Endocrinology for the House Officer

Endocrinology for the House Officer

Warner M. Burch, M.D.
Departments of Medicine and Pharmacology
Duke University Medical Center
Durham, North Carolina

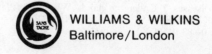

WILLIAMS & WILKINS
Baltimore/London

Editor: James L. Sangston
Associate Editor: Jonathan W. Pine, Jr.
Design: Bob Och
Production: Carol Eckhart

Copyright ©, 1984
Williams & Wilkins
428 East Preston Street
Baltimore, MD 21202, U.S.A.

Made in the United States of America

Library of Congress Cataloging in Publication Data

Burch, Warner M.
 Endocrinology for the house officer.
 Includes index.
  1. Endocrine glands—Diseases. 2. Clinical endocrinology. I. Title. [DNLM: 1. Endocrine diseases. 2. Endocrine glands. WK 100 B947e]
RC648.B87 1984   616.4   83-23479
ISBN 0-683-01132-4

Composed and printed at the
Waverly Press, Inc.
Mt. Royal and Guilford Aves.
Baltimore, MD 21202, U.S.A.

Endocrinology for the House Officer addresses endocrine problems commonly encountered in medical practice. Its approach is largely problem-oriented with emphasis on workup, diagnosis, and treatment. It is not intended to be a textbook of endocrinology but a convenient and practical "how to" and "why" source that can be used on the wards and in the clinic.

Warner M. Burch, M.D.

Acknowledgments

Francis A. Neelon, M.D., reviewed and copy-edited this book. His comments and sage advice helped immensely. Thank you, Frank. My family deserves recognition for their support. I love you: Vivian, Pweebe, Greta, Marcus, Joshua, and Seth.

Contents

Chapter 1

Endocrine Tests

Probably nothing is more confusing than the myriad of endocrine studies available to the house officer. There are numerous studies but only those which are widely available will be discussed in this chapter. As with any laboratory study, one must have a clinical diagnosis or suspicion from the history or physical exam that leads one to order a particular study. What to do with the laboratory results can be a problem. When there is discordance between the clinical diagnosis and the lab results which "don't fit," then most often it is the laboratory that is in error. Somehow clinicians have been "sold a bill of goods" regarding the infallibility of a laboratory result. If your clinical diagnosis seems firm and yet the lab says something else, then call the laboratory; ask for a repeat run; check to see if the proper patient sample was assayed; how good was that assay?; etc. With endocrine studies in general, it is very important that you know the quality and reliability of the laboratory to which the specimen was sent. This point cannot be overemphasized.

THYROID TESTS

Serum Thyroxine (T4): The most widely used method for measuring total serum T4 is the radioimmunoassay (RIA). It is reliable, inexpensive, and specific. Normal serum T4(RIA) levels range between 5 and 12 ug/dl. Serum T4 is affected by two major factors: thyroidal secretion of T4 and the serum binding capacity for T4. Since > 99.9% of the T4 circulating is bound to protein, any alteration in the binding capacity as well as in T4 secretion leads to abnormal serum T4 levels. To accurately interpret the level of T4 one also needs to know about the serum T4 binding capacity. The following case illustrates a common situation: A 24 yr-old woman was referred because of symptoms of anxiety and rapid heart rate; her serum T4(RIA) 14.5 ug/dl (normal 5-12). She was taking an oral contraceptive. On physical exam the pulse was 95 and no goiter was palpated. Is this hyperthyroidism? Unlikely, but what one really needs is a measure of the serum T4 binding capacity since estrogens increase thyroid binding globulin (TBG), the major T4 binding serum protein. The T4 binding capacity of serum is assessed by measuring the T3U.

<u>T3U or T3 Resin Uptake:</u>   The T3U measures indirectly the number of unoccupied protein binding sites for T4 and T3 in serum.   The test gets its name from the radiolabeled T3 which is used the <u>in vitro</u> assay. Radiolabeled T3 is added to the patient's serum and competes for binding sites on the TBG molecule. Radiolabeled T3 is used instead of T4 because the the assay time is shorter. A resin or some other inert material is then added to adsorb any unbound radiolabeled T3.   The radioactivity of the resin is then counted and expressed as per cent of total counts added to the assay tube.

Schematically the T3U assay is performed as follows:

```
|--
|--
|--T4
|--
|--T4
```

represents the TBG molecule with T4 bound to several binding sites;

T3* represents radiolabeled T3; and   [ ]   the <u>resin</u> which

is later counted for radioactivity yielding the T3U:

```
|--
|--T4        T3*  T3*                        |--T3*
|--     +    T3*  T3*  -----> add resin ---> |--T4    +  | T3*    |
|--          T3*  T3*                        |--T3*       | T3* T3* |
|--T4                                        |--T3*
                                             |--T4
```
                                             T3U normal

If the sites on TBG are under-occupied by T4 (as in hypothyroidism with decreased T4 secretion), then more radiolabeled T3 will bind to the protein and less radiolabel T3 will be adsorbed to the resin. Thus, the T3U will be low. Schematically the T3U assay of hypothyroid serum would be as follows:

```
|--
|--T4        T3*  T3*                        |--T3*
|--     +    T3*  T3*  -----> add resin ---> |--T4    +  | T3* T3* |
|--          T3*  T3*                        |--T3
|--                                          |--T3*
                                             |--T3*
```
                                             T3U low

In patients with hyperthyroidism (increased T4 secretion), the T3U is elevated since most of the sites on TBG are occupied by T4 so that less radiolabeled T3 can be bound by the protein and more to the resin. Schematically the T3U assay would look like this:

```
|--T4
|--T4         T3* T3*
|--      +    T3* T3*    -----> add resin ---->
|--T4         T3* T3*
|--T4
```
```
|--T4
|--T4        ┌ T3*──┐
|--T3*  +    │ T3* T3* │
|--T4        └ T3*-T3*─┘
|--T4
```

                                        T3U high

The normal range of values for the T3U depends on the particular type of resin used which means various labs have different normal ranges for T3U. In all cases, however, the T3U is inversely proportional to the number of unoccupied binding sites on TBG (low T3U--high TBG; high T3U--low TBG).

When TBG levels are raised (i.e., more binding sites for radiolabel T3, less radioactivity for resin to adsorb), the T3U will be low. The most frequent medication that raises TBG is estrogen. The T3U assay in this situation is diagrammed as follows:

```
|--    |--
|--T4  |--         T3* T3*
|--    |--    +    T3* T3*    -----> add resin ---->
|--    |--T4       T3* T3*
|--T4  |--T4
```
```
|--T3*  |--T3*      ┌────┐
|--T4   |--T3*      │ T3* │
|--T3*  |--     +   │ T3* │
|--     |--T4       └────┘
|--T4   |--T4
```

                                        low T3U

The patient mentioned above who was taking an oral contraceptive did have raised TBG levels which accounted for the elevated serum T4 and this was confirmed with a low T3U. There are numerous factors that may affect TBG and thus the T3U value. These factors are listed in the following table.

Increased TBG	Decreased TBG
Estrogen therapy	Androgen therapy
Pregnancy	Severe hypoproteinemia
Acute hepatitis	Chronic liver disease
Acute intermittent porphyria	Glucocorticoid excess
Hereditary TBG increase	Hereditary TBG deficiency
	Acromegaly
T3U low	T3U high

Some medications, such as salicylates (high doses), dilantin, and clofibrate, compete with T4 to bind on TBG. This leads to high T3U values but also to lower T4(RIA) levels. It should be remembered that the T3U has nothing to do with the serum levels of T3.

To correct for variation in TBG (and therefore the T4 and T3U values), a calculated value called the Free Thyroid Index (FTI) may be used. The FTI is an attempt to normalize discordant serum T4 and T3U values and is the product of the T4(RIA) times the T3U. This calculated number correlates well with the levels of free T4 and thus is named Free Thyroid Index.

Free Thyroxine (FT4): The unbound or free thyroxine (FT4) is the metabolically active hormone fraction. It accounts for less than 0.1% of the total T4 circulating in the blood. Ideally, the measurement of the free T4 would eliminate most of the confusion regarding binding protein abnormalities because it circulates within well-defined limits in the euthyroid patient. However, free T4 levels are not routinely available because the measurement of this small quantity of unbound T4 is technically difficult, time-consuming, and requires dialysis techniques for accurate quantitation. The commercial kits for measurement of free T4 determinations are not totally reliable. Because of these factors and the availability of serum T4 and T3U measurements, the FT4 is rarely used clinically.

T3(RIA): The primary hormone secreted and the major circulating thyroid hormone is thyroxine (T4). However, T4 is rapidly deiodinated into triiodothyronine (T3) by 5'-deiodinase found in many tissues but especially in the liver. T3 is the metabolically active thyroid hormone which binds to nuclear receptors of target tissues. T3 circulates in the blood but at concentrations 50 times lower than T4. Radioimmunoassays of T3 are specific and are generally available. Serum T3(RIA) levels range between 90 and 190 ng/dl. T3 is also bound to TBG but the affinity is less avid. Nevertheless, serum T3(RIA) measurements are subject to the same limitations regarding protein binding as with T4 determinations [e.g., estrogens increase TBG and therefore T3(RIA) levels]. Serum T3(RIA) levels are elevated in hyperthyroidism, often to a greater degree than the T4(RIA). Serum T3(RIA) is useful in iodine deficient states where the T4 may be low yet T3 normal. T3(RIA) is particularly useful in hyperthyroid states such as toxic nodular goiter where the serum T4(RIA) may be normal.

Thyroid Stimulating Hormone (TSH): TSH is a glycoprotein secreted by the pituitary. The rate of TSH production is dependent on the levels of free thyroxine and is regulated by a classical negative feedback system: Low levels of T4 lead to TSH secretion which stimulates thyroid hormone production and release which in turn decreases pituitary TSH output. Conversely, high T4 or T3 levels suppress TSH secretion. Serum TSH is measured by radioimmunoassay with normal ranges from 0-6 uU/ml. Most TSH assays are not sensitive enough to tell the difference between 0 and 2 uU/ml. Although TSH levels are low in hyperthyroidism, the sensitivity of the assay does not allow differentiation between euthyroid and hyperthyroid subjects. The serum TSH is elevated in primary hypothyroidism reaching levels > 100 uU/ml. If there is a question of primary hypothyroidism clinically, serum TSH determination is extremely helpful.

Thyrotropin Releasing Hormone (TRH): TRH is a tripeptide secreted by the hypothalmus and circulated to the pituitary via the portal-hypophyseal capillary system. TRH stimulates the certain pituitary cells called thyrotropes to secrete TSH. If ambient levels of T4 or T3 are high, then the thyrotrope will not respond to TRH with a rise in TSH. In primary hypothyroidism in which the TSH is already elevated, TRH will greatly augment the release of TSH. TRH administration is extremely useful clinically in states which hyperthyroidism is suspected and the diagnosis is not clear using static determinations such as T4(RIA), T3U, and T3(RIA). Giving TRH provides a dynamic test which assesses the functional integrity of the thyrotrope. The TRH study is performed as follows:

Blood is drawn for baseline TSH (0 time). TRH (protirelin) 500 ug is given iv over 15-20 sec and blood drawn again at 30 min for TSH determination. TSH levels peak normally around 20-30 min post TRH. The normal response is dependent upon age and sex. Females generally have at least 6 uU/ml rise above the basal level. Males < 40 yrs of age should have a similar rise (> 6 uU/ml) whereas males > 40 should have at least a 2 uU/ml rise.

In primary hypothyroidism the response to TRH is increased. Hyperthyroid patients, patients with euthyroid Graves' disease, or subjects taking excessive doses of replacement thyroid (T4 or T3) or pharmacological amounts of glucocorticoid will not have a rise in serum TSH. In patients suspected of having hyperthyroidism the TRH study has nearly replaced the use of exogenous thyroid hormone to see whether radioiodine uptake is suppressed or not.

Thyroidal 24-hr Radioactive Iodine Uptake: The thyroid
gland concentrates iodine which it uses for thyroxine
production.   Because the thyroid acts as a sump for iodine
and relative little iodine is trapped anywhere else in the
body, the uptake of radioactive iodine (RAI) is a useful
marker of thyroid function. The source of radioactivity has
traditionally been 131-Iodine. The RAI uptake is calculated
as the percentage of total administered radioactivity taken
up by the thyroid.   This determination is usually made 24
hrs after an oral ingestion of tracer doses of I-131 (6-8
uCi). The normal 24-hr RAI uptake is 10-30%.

If the thyroid is not functioning (e.g., hypothyroidism
or in subacute thyroiditis where the follicular cell cannot
concentrate iodine), then the 24-hr RAI uptake is low.

If the iodine content of the plasma pool is elevated
secondary to ingestion of iodine-rich foods (kelp) or
medications (saturated solution of potassium iodide, Ornade,
Amiodarone, etc.) or secondary to the administration of
radiographic agents, the 24-hr value for tracer uptake will
be low even though the thyroid may have perfectly normal
function.

In a diffuse toxic goiter the thyroidal trapping of
iodine is increased, and the 24-hr I-131 uptake will be
elevated. 123-Iodine is now a frequent source of radioactive
iodine since there is less radiation exposure to the
thyroid.   The amount of radiation delivered to the thyroid
by I-131 is approximately 1.5 rad/uCi (assuming normal size
gland and 20% 24-hr uptake) which is 100 times the radiation
exposure of I-123 (0.015 rad/uCi). All radionuclide tests
are contra-indicated during pregnancy.

Thyroid Imaging or Scan: Imaging of the thyroid is possible
by utilizing radionuclides.   These are useful in
ascertaining whether a particular area of the thyroid such
as a nodule is functioning, that is, is it able to trap and
concentrate the radionuclide?   The most often used
radiotracers are technetium-99m pertechnetate, I-131, and
I-123.   TcO4-99m (5 mCi) is administrated iv and thyroid
imaging is performed within 30 min. TcO4-99m assesses only
the transport ability of the follicular cells whereas iodine
radionuclides assess both transport and organification of
iodine to thyroglobulin. The amount of radiation delivered
to the thyroid is 0.2 rad/mCi TcO4-99m. I-131 (50 uCi) is
administrated po and the scan performed 24 hrs later. The
thyroid scan with pertechnetate is more convenient for the
patient and also has considerable less thyroidal radiation
(i.e., 1 rad vs 75 rads for I-131). I-123 may also be used
for imaging but this is not always available because of its
short half-life (13 hrs).

PITUITARY TESTS

<u>Growth Hormone:</u>   Growth hormone is measured in three circumstances: 1) when there is clinical evidence of <u>acromegaly or gigantism;</u> 2) when there is evidence of <u>growth failure</u> (e.g., short stature); 3) when it is necessary to ascertain whether there is <u>adequate pituitary reserve</u> since the function of pituitary somatotrope is very sensitive to mass lesions (e.g., tumors, cysts). Growth hormone (GH) is assayed in serum or plasma using radioimmunoassay. A single determination of GH can be useful in few cases, but often dynamic studies (stimulation or suppression tests) are necessary.

If the question is <u>acromegaly,</u> then a single sample drawn after the patient fasted overnight and at bedrest in which the GH is > 10 ng/ml is highly suggestive of acromegaly. Any form of stress (exercise, surgery, smoking, etc.) will raise GH and thus caution must be taken on borderline elevated values. Acromegaly is usually confirmed using an oral glucose tolerance test (GTT) [see Diabetes Mellitus, page 36]. Blood is obtained at 0, 60, 120, and 180 min for GH determination. Since rises in blood glucose suppress GH levels in healthy patients, normal subjects will exhibit a decrease in GH to < 2 ng/ml within two hours. Up to a third of acromegalic patients will have a paradoxical rise in the GH levels during the GTT.

If the question is <u>growth hormone deficiency,</u> then a single determination using any form of stress to raise GH may be all that is necessary. In children blood drawn for GH 90 minutes after sleep is helpful since GH is secreted during REM sleep. However a more practical study is to have the child exercise (run up and down steps for 15 minutes) and then draw blood for GH level. Any values > 5 ng/ml excludes GH deficiency. A variety of stimulatory tests are available to raise GH levels. When to order these studies and how to interpret them requires discernment. In children with short stature and low GH value after exercise or in the patient with possible hypopituitism, a stimulatory test is indicated.

The "gold standard" study is insulin-induced hypoglycemia which produces a profound stress reaction that is followed by GH release as well as ACTH and subsequent rise in serum cortisol.

The <u>insulin-induced hypoglycemia test (IIHT)</u> is performed in the AM after an overnight fast with the patient at bedrest. An indwelling needle in the forearm is recommended so that multiple samples can be obtained. Blood for basal levels of GH and cortisol is taken at -15 and 0 mins. Regular insulin (0.1 U/kg for normal size patients and 0.15-0.2 U/kg for patients with insulin resistance, e.g., obesity) is injected rapidly intravenously. If there is clinical evidence of hypopituitarism, then a lower dose of insulin is used (0.05 U/kg) since profound hypoglycemia is more likely. Plasma glucose is measured at 0, 15, 30, 45, and 60 min. A decrease of the plasma glucose to 50% of baseline value or < 40 mg/dl is considered an adequate hypoglycemic response which is necessary to interpret the GH and cortisol levels. Blood for GH and cortisol is measured at 0, 30, 60, and 90 min. Dextrose (50%) should be available to treat severe hypoglycemia (e.g. obtundation, seizure).

After hypoglycemia is assured (hunger, palpitations, perspiration), the patient may drink fruit juice to decrease symptoms if necessary. The nadir for the blood sugar is usually 20-30 min with rises of GH and cortisol later (fig. 1.1).

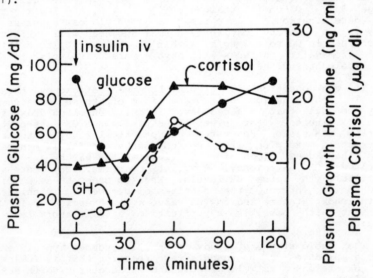

Figure 1.1   The response of plasma growth hormone and cortisol to insulin-induced hypoglycemia.

Even though sugar may have to be given iv or po, continue to draw blood at the indicated intervals. GH levels normally rise to > 9 ng/ml 60-90 min post insulin injection. The

disadvantages of insulin-induced hypoglycemia are obvious:
close monitoring of the patient is a necessity; hypoglycemia
is uncomfortable and potential problems very real; it is not
easily performed in children; and one must be sure of
adequate hypoglycemia (stress) to have a valid study. In
addition up to 20% of normal subjects have an impaired or
absent GH response to this "gold standard." Patients with
obesity, Cushing's syndrome, and chronic renal failure may
also have an impaired or absent GH response. However, a
normal response excludes GH deficiency.

Other growth hormone stimulatory studies include oral
L-dopa and arginine infusion for adults, and oral clonidine
and intramuscular glucagon for children.

Adrenocorticotropic Hormone (ACTH or corticotropin): Since
there are abundant numbers of corticotrope cells dispersed
throughout the pituitary, ACTH is generally the last tropic
hormone lost in pituitary disease. Assessing the pituitary-
adrenal axis begins with measuring baseline 24 hr urine for
either 17-hydroxycorticosteroids (17-OHCS) or free cortisol
(UC). The products of the adrenal glands are measured since
determinations of ACTH are not readily available nor as
reliable as one needs. Normal urinary 17-OHCS levels range
between 2 and 6.5 mg/gm creatinine. UC values depend upon
the method and the specificity of the antibody. Thus, normal
ranges must be established in each laboratory.

Normal ACTH levels range between 20 and 80 pg/ml. The
method of collection and handling of the plasma sample is
critical. Since ACTH adheres to glass avidly, blood must be
collected, stored on ice, centrifuged within 30 min
(preferably earlier), and then the plasma stored at -20° C
in polypropylene vials. Assaying the ACTH is technically
difficult and time consuming. The reliability of the
laboratory must be impeccable. Plasma ACTH levels are
useful in separating the types of Cushing's syndrome
particularly in ectopic ACTH where levels are often very high
(> 200 pg/ml) and in adrenal adenoma where ACTH levels are
non-measurable.

Stimulatory tests to indirectly evaluate ACTH reserve
include insulin-induced hypoglycemia test and metyrapone
loading. The information gained from these studies is
helpful in deciding whether patients have pituitary disease
or whether those with known pituitary dysfunction (e.g.,
after pituitary surgery) will need long-term glucocorticoid
coverage.

Hypoglycemia is a potent stress. Utilizing the insulin-induced hypoglycemia study (IIHT) is an excellent method to gather GH and cortisol data to assess the integrity of the pituitary-adrenal axis. Plasma cortisols are measured at the intervals listed above in the insulin-induced hypoglycemia test. Plasma cortisol should rise at least 10 ug/dl to a value > 20 ug/dl in normal subjects (Fig. 1.1). This study assumes the adrenal glands can function to respond to ACTH. Since hypoglycemia is potential life-threatening to the hypoadrenal patient, one should avoid this study in patients with known Addison's disease.

Metyrapone inhibits the final enzymatic step (11-beta-hydroxylase) in the synthesis of cortisol. This leads to a build up of 11-deoxycortisol, the immediate precursor of cortisol and to a decrease in cortisol production. The fall in serum cortisol levels is sensed by the pituitary corticotropes. The corticotropes respond by increasing ACTH production in the classical negative feedback loop. Although serum deoxycortisol levels rise, the pituitary does not recognize deoxycortisol as a glucocorticoid hormone. As a result, in normal subjects administration of metyrapone leads to elevated levels of deoxycortisol and low, normal or raised serum cortisol concentrations (the absolute levels of cortisol depend upon the effectiveness of the metyrapone-induced blockade).

Metyrapone is usually administered orally using either of the two following protocols: an abbreviated overnight study or the classic 3-day study.

In the overnight study, metyrapone (3 gm or 30 mg/kg) is taken at bedtime with milk to avoid gastric irritation. Since metyrapone will decrease serum cortisol at the time (early AM) when the corticotrope is most sensitive to falling cortisol levels, there is an exaggerated ACTH output which leads to elevated levels of serum deoxycortisol. At 7-8 AM blood is drawn for deoxycortisol and cortisol levels. The normal response is > 7 ug/dl for serum deoxycortisol. Serum cortisol levels should be low (< 5 ug/dl) to assure metyrapone produced an adequate blockade. If there is a normal deoxycortisol response, no further study is needed to assess the pituitary-adrenal axis.

If abnormal, then the 3-day protocol is performed because it is the "gold standard" of the metyrapone studies. Urine is collected for 24 hrs as baseline for determination of 17-OHCS (day 1). Metyrapone is given 750 mg every 4 hrs po for 6 doses (day 2).

Again metyrapone blocks cortisol production which in turn normally stimulates ACTH and deoxycortisol production. Since both cortisol and deoxycortisol have the 17,21-dihydroxyl,20-keto groups which are measured as Porter-Silber chromatogens in the 17-OHCS assay, urine 17-OHCS levels should rise. A 24-hr urine is collected on the 3rd day (day following oral metyrapone). A normal rise in urine 17-OHCS is 2.5 to 3 times the baseline day's 17-OHCS value. It is also useful to obtain plasma cortisol and deoxycortisol at 7-8 AM on day 2 and day 3 following metyrapone to assess adequacy of the metyrapone-blockade. A sample protocol orders for this study is given below:

1) DAY 1--Collect 24 hr urine (7 AM-7 AM) for 17-OHCS

2) DAY 2--Blood draw at 7 AM for plasma cortisol and
         deoxycortisol
         Metryapone 750 mg q 4 hr po times 6 doses
         (Start giving medication at 8 AM)
         Collect 24 hr urine (7 AM-7 AM) for 17-OHCS

3) DAY 3--Blood draw at 7 AM for plasma cortisol and
         deoxycortisol
         Collect 24 hr urine (7 AM-7 AM) for 17-OHCS

We measure 17-OHCS level on the day after metyrapone since the last two doses of metyrapone given on the 2nd day produce the lowest cortisol levels (early AM) which stimulate ACTH and thus steroidogenesis reflected in the large amount of 17-OHCS in the subsequent collection. It is important not to give any exogenous glucocorticoid (small doses of dexamethasone) "to cover" the patient during any metyrapone study since this will inhibit ACTH release (as cortisol does), and therefore no effect on adreno-steroidogenesis will be seen.

Both insulin-induced hypoglycemia and metyrapone blockade are artificial forms of stress. Though ACTH reserve may be adequate by these studies, the question remains whether patients can handle stress in real situation (severe infections, myocardial infarction, major surgery, etc). Generally, if one of these studies demonstrates adequate ACTH-cortisol reserve, then no steroid coverage is necessary.

Dexamethasone suppression studies are done whenever there is evidence of glucocorticoid excess (obesity, hypertension, protein catabolism, etc.) and the patient is not taking exogenous steroids (the most common cause of Cushing's syndrome). The study is based on the observation that small doses of a potent glucocorticosteroid (dexamethasone) can inhibit the normal pituitary corticotrope so that no ACTH is released (the typical negative feedback loop) and thus there is decreased production of cortisol. Since the amount of dexamethasone does not interfere with the assay of cortisol or 17-OHCS, there is a fall of serum cortisol which is reflected in low urine cortisol and urine 17-OHCS levels. There are several ways to administer the dexamethasone.

A short overnight study is very useful in the outpatient setting to assess whether there is glucocorticoid excess (Cushing's syndrome). Dexamethasone 1 mg is taken between 11 PM and midnight, and a serum cortisol drawn between 8 and 9 AM the following morning. This level should be < 5 ug/dl. If the serum cortisol is > 5 ug/ml, then a variety of possibilities exist: Cushing's syndrome; patient did not take dexamethasone; stress during the night; traffic rush getting to clinic; patient is pregnant or taking meds such as estrogens which increase cortisol binding globulin; the patient is taking anticonvulsant drugs which speed the metabolism of dexamethasone so that adequate suppressive levels are not reached; severe mental depression; and obesity.

A 24-hr urine for cortisol determination should be collected (see Adrenal Tests) if the plasma cortisol does not suppress with overnight dexamethasone. If the UC is elevated, then the diagnosis of hypercortisolism is confirmed and a protocol using Liddle's criteria for differentiating the categories of Cushing's syndrome is necessary.

This classic study is performed as follows: Two baseline 24-hr urines are collected for 17-OHCS and UC (days 1 & 2). Normal urine 17-OHCS is < 6.5 mg/gm creatinine and UC < 100 ug/24 hr. Dexamethasone 0.5 mg is given po q 6 hr times 8 doses (days 3 & 4) and a 24-hr urine is collected on day 4 for 17-OHCS and UC. This amount of dexamethasone (low dose; 2 mg/day) will suppress the normal corticotrope, but in patients with Cushing's syndrome (any state of hypercortisolism) the 24-hr urine will not suppress to < 2.5 mg 17-OHCS/gm creatinine or < 25 ug cortisol/24 hr. In Cushing's disease (pituitary-dependent adrenal hyperplasia) the abnormal corticotropes in the pituitary adenoma are sensitive to glucocorticoid inhibition only at much higher doses of dexamethasone. Thus, dexamethasone 2.0 mg is given po q 6 hr times 8 doses (days 5 & 6) and a 24-hr urine collected on day 6 for 17-OHCS determination. With this high dose of dexamethasone (8 mg/day) patients with Cushing's disease have urine 17-OHCS < 50% of baseline values of days 1 & 2, whereas patients with hypercortisolism due to adrenal adenoma/carcinoma or ectopic ACTH syndrome will have no suppression of the 17-OHCS. The reliability of the > 50% criteria for suppression in Cushing's disease is somewhat arbitrary since some patients with Cushing's disease may only suppress 35%. The point is there is significant lowering of urine 17-OHCS with high dose dexamethasone in pituitary-dependent adrenal hyperplasia.

Others have used modifications of the high dose dexamethaxone study to shorten the workup. At 8 AM a baseline plasma cortisol is drawn and at 11 PM 8.0 mg of dexamethasone is given po. At 8 AM the next morning plasma cortisol measured. Patients with Cushing's disease have plasma cortisol level < 50% of baseline value. Do not confuse this high dose dexamethasone study with the overnight study (1.0 mg of dexamethasone) used to screen patients for Cushing's syndrome.

<u>Thyroid Stimulating Hormone (TSH) or Thyrotropin:</u> Serum TSH levels are elevated in primary hypothyroidism, however serum TSH determinations cannot distinquish normal from low values (page 5). If hypothyroidism is suspected on basis of pituitary disease, then there are usually signs and symptoms to suggest loss of other tropic hormones. Isolated TSH deficiency is a rarity. Pituitary disease is likely when the T4 and T3U values are low and the TSH is "normal." In cases of suspected hyperthyroidism, the TRH study (see page 5) is very helpful since TSH levels fail to rise when TRH is given to hyperthyroid patients. In primary hypothyroidism TRH produces an exaggerated rise in the serum TSH. TRH does not raise serum GH levels in normal subjects. TRH does stimulate a rise in serum prolactin of at least 3 times basal value to a peak > 20 ng/ml. In 70-80 % of acromegalics, TRH stimulates GH levels to rise (often 10 to 30 times baseline), a finding that has been as reliable as the use of the oral GTT in making the diagnosis of acromegaly. The TRH study has also been used to follow patients having received therapy for acromegaly to assess how treatment modified the course of their disease.

<u>Follicular Stimulating Hormone (FSH) and Luteinizing Hormone (LH):</u> Serum FSH and LH levels vary depending on method and standards used. The most reliable assays are those utilizing RIA techniques. If the standard Second IRP/HMG is used, the FSH in postpubertal females range between 4 to 15 mIU/ml in the follicular and luteal phases and between 10 and 50 mIU/ml at midcycle. Postmenopausal females, females with primary ovarian failure (e.g., surgical removal, Turner's syndrome), and males with primary hypogonadism will

have elevated values (40-350 mIU/ml). LH levels in the female again vary with the phase within the menstrual cycle: follicular (4-30 mIU/ml); midcycle (30-150 mIU/ml); and luteal (4 to 40 mIU/ml). LH levels are raised in the postmenopausal female and in the postpubertal patients with primary hypogonadism (> 40 mIU/ml).

If there is a question of hypopituitarism in a postmenopausal female, one should measure the serum FSH and LH. Finding elevated serum gonadotropins (which is normal and appropiate for estrogen deficit state) weigh strongly against the possibility of hypopituitarism. Gonadotropin releasing hormone (GnRH or gonadorelin) is available to be used in a few select patients with secondary hypogonadism and in an occasional patient in whom there is a question of whether the pituitary gonadotropes are functioning normally. GnRH (100 ug) is given iv and blood is drawn at 0, 15, 30, and 60 min. LH response to GnRH is greater than FSH and normally rises to values between 25 and 80 mIU/ml by 30 min. An intact response can exclude gonadotrope dysfunction, but an impaired or absent response cannot be used to define the anatomic abnormality (pituitary vs hypothalmus).

Prolactin: Prolactin is secreted by the pituitary lacto-trope. The lactotrope is under tonic inhibition by a hypothalmic substance called prolactin inhibitory factor (PIF) which is probably dopamine. Prolactin is measured by RIA. The upper limit of normal is 20 ng/ml for females and 15 ng/ml for males. The lower limits of detectability in the prolactin RIA do not distinquish between low and normal prolactin levels (similar to TSH determinations). Serum prolactin is elevated in many situations. Females with amenorrhea/oligomenorrhea or galactorrhea and males with impotence as well as patients with suspected or known pituitary tumor need to have their serum prolactin measured. Prolactin produces hypogonadism by several mechanisms leading to low estrogen levels in females and testosterone deficiency in males. Prolactin inhibits the pulsatile secretion of GnRH necessary for the midcycle LH surge and inhibits the positive feedback of estrogen on gonadotropin secretion. Very high levels of prolactin may directly inhibit gonadal function.

Prolactinomas (prolactin-secreting pituitary adenomas) may produce serum levels of prolactin > 1000 ng/ml. Other causes of hyperprolactinemia include nursing postpartum mothers, functional hyperprolactinemia (no identifiable pituitary tumor), hypothalmic disorders such as sarcoidosis, histiocytosis, parasellar tumors, and stalk lesions (all presumably decrease PIF which releases the lactotrope to secrete prolactin), and pharmacological agents that decrease monoamines or monoamine action (that is, lower dopamine, the putative PIF). These drugs include methyldopa, reserpine, phenothiazines, tricyclic antidepressants, and narcotics. Patients with primary hypothyroidism (TRH stimulates prolactin secretion) and patients with chest wall diseases and spinal cord lesions (tactile stimulation of nipple areola will stimulate prolactin release) may have elevated serum prolactin levels. Subjects with chronic renal failure may have serum prolactin levels up to 150 ng/ml which return to normal after transplantation but not with dialysis.

Dehydration test: The dehydration study is used in the evaluation of polyuria and polydipsia. Most often the differential diagnosis is among neurogenic diabetes insipidus, nephrogenic diabetes insipidus, or primary polydipsia (psychogenic or compulsive water drinker). Diabetes mellitus is easily excluded by identifying glycosuria and elevated blood sugar.

Plasma osmolality (largely determined by the serum sodium concentration) is the primary stimulant of vasopressin release. As plasma osmolality rises, osmoreceptors in the hypothalmus signal adjacent neurons of the supraoptic and paraventricular nuclei to release vasopressin which is stored in the distal axons of these nuclei terminating in the pituitary stalk and posterior pituitary gland. Vasopressin or antidiuretic hormone (ADH) levels are available in only a few centers so dehydration is used as the biological assay to assess the action of ADH on the kidney. ADH concentrates urine by decreasing free water clearance. In the absence of ADH, urine is dilute and its osmolality low.

Normal (ad lib water) plasma osmolality ranges between 270 and 290 mOsm/kg. If the plasma osmolality and serum sodium are > 295 mOsm/kg and > 143 meq/l respectively under conditions of ad lib fluid intake, the diagnosis of primary polydipsia is excluded.

The dehydration test must be carefully performed and the patient closely monitored. If the history suggests significant polyuria, then total fluid restriction is begun at 7-8 AM after baseline body weight and urine and plasma osmolality are determined. In cases of less severe polyuria total fluid restriction may begin earlier (hs) after the same baseline variables are measured. A flow sheet is used to record responses and should have the following headings: body weight, urine specific gravity (a convenient bedside monitor of urine osmolality), urine volume, urine and plasma osmolality. Body weight and urine values are assessed hourly. When the urine osmolality stabilizes (specific gravity unchanged at the bedside and the lab confirms that the hourly increase in urine osmolality < 30 mOsm/kg for 3 hours), then blood is drawn for plasma osmolality. A plasma value > 288 mOsm/kg assures adequate dehydration. Some patients will surreptitiously imbibe water during the study and thus will not concentrate their urine. After urine osmolality stabilizes, aqueous vasopressin 5 units is given sc and urine and plasma osmolality are measured one hour later. If body weight decreases below 3% of the initial weight, then the test is stopped after the plasma and urine osmolalities are measured and the response to aqueous vasopressin performed.

In patients with neurogenic diabetes insipidus the urine osmolality will rise > 150 mOsm/kg after vasopressin is given. Normal subjects and those with nephrogenic diabetes insipidus will not have a rise in urine osmolality in response to vasopressin. Some difficulty in interpreting this test arises in those patients with diabetes insipidus who have residual capacity to secrete ADH under hypertonic conditions of the dehydration test and in compulsive water drinkers who have diluted the concentration gradient in the renal medulla such that even high levels of ADH cannot produce a normally concentrated urine during the short interval of this test. In these circumstances the clinical assessment is important. If there is still doubt regarding the diagnosis, then the plasma from the dehydration test should be assayed for vasopressin. In diabetes insipidus (neurogenic) the plasma vasopressin will be low whereas vasopressin levels will be appropiately elevated in primary polydipsia.

ADRENAL TESTS

The adrenal glands secrete a variety of hormones: cortisol, aldosterone, and adrenal androgens from the adrenal cortex; and epinephrine and norepinephrine from the adrenal medulla. Of these hormones the glucocorticoid, cortisol, is the most important for sustaining life.

Glucocorticoids: The synthesis and secretion of cortisol is regulated by ACTH with the most frequent pulsations of ACTH coming between 6 and 8 AM. This accounts for the circadian variation of serum cortisol, with the highest levels occurring around 8 AM (15-25 ug/dl) and the lowest levels between 11 PM and 4 AM (< 5 ug/dl). The spontaneous rhythm of cortisol release can be altered by psychological stresses (e.g., mental preparation for major surgery, athletic competition, or college exams) and <u>physical stresses</u> (e.g., severe illness, surgery, trauma, fever, severe dehydration, or hypoglycemia) as well as <u>changing time schelude</u> (e.g., work nights and sleep in the daytime). A major stress such as cardiac surgery can increase cortisol production six-fold. This does not mean the serum cortisol concentration will rise six-fold. Cortisol is a steroid which is insoluble in aqueous solutions and circulates bound to plasma proteins, the major one called <u>cortisol binding globulin (CBG).</u> CBG acts as sump and buffer such that a six-fold rise in cortisol secretion may be reflected as a two- or three-fold rise in serum cortisol. Cortisol is nearly totally (90%) bound to CBG up to concentrations of 25 ug/dl, but as cortisol concentrations rise above this level the binding capacity of CBG is exceeded and the proportion of unbound or free cortisol rises greatly. For example, when the total serum cortisol is 40 ug/dl, then the concentration of free cortisol is 10 times higher (10 ug/dl) than when the total serum cortisol is 10 ug/dl (1 ug/dl).

The synthesis of CBG is <u>increased by estrogens, oral</u> <u>contraceptives, pregnancy, and hyperthyroidism</u> leading to elevated levels of CBG, and thus, raised serum cortisol concentrations. This is important to remember when trying to suppress plasma cortisol with dexamethasone. A woman taking an oral contraceptive may not have a fall in serum cortisol after an overnight dose of dexamethasone. CBG levels can be elevated on a familial basis as well. CBG levels are decreased with hypothyroidism, liver disease, nephrotic syndrome, and multiple myeloma. Despite changes in CBG concentrations, the free or unbound cortisol remains normal as long as the pituitary-adrenal axis is normal.

A fraction of the 8 to 25 mg of cortisol normally secreted by the adrenals each day is found in the urine as free cortisol (UC; < 100 mg/24 hrs). The actual values for normal UC must be established for each laboratory since extraction and specificity of the antibody vary. UC is a reliable means of assessing the adrenal glucocorticoid status especially when there is a question of cortisol excess. UC determination is generally preerable to 17-OHCS for several reasons: UC values correlate well with cortisol production rates; UC is measured by RIA and is not subject to color interference which often occurs in the 17-OHCS assay when patients take drugs. In addition, 17-OHCS measures end-products and intermediates of cortisol metabolism. Normal urine 17-OHCS levels range between 2.0 and 6.5 mg/gm creatinine.

<u>Stimulatory studies</u> of cortisol are necessary in patients suspected of adrenal insufficiency. Numerous tests have been used to assess adrenal reserve; the type of study

depends on the clinical situation. Often the circumstance may not warrant a provocative study. If the plasma cortisol is elevated in a stress situation (e.g., trauma septicemia, etc), then stimulatory studies are unnecessary since the pituitary-adrenal axis is intact.

If the index of suspicion is low (weak, tired, normally pigmented subject in whom one wishes to rule out Addison's disease), then a short ACTH (Cortrosyn) study is ideal.

Blood for plasma cortisol is drawn (0 time). Synthetic 1-24 ACTH (cosyntropin; Cortrosyn) 0.25 mg is given intramuscularly (or intravenously). Another plasma cortisol is obtained at 45 min since the maximal rise in plasma cortisol occurs between 30 and 60 min.

Normal stimulation is > 7 ug/dl above 0 time and often there is 15 to 20 ug/dl rise. This study is particularly useful in the out-patient setting. A normal response excludes the diagnosis of primary adrenal insufficiency.

If the cortisol fails to increase with the short Cortrosyn study, then a formal inpatient study is necessary to confirm the diagnosis of primary or secondary adrenal insufficiency.

A 24 hr urine is collected as baseline for 17-OHCS and/or UC. Cortrosyn, 0.25 mg, in 500 ml of saline is infused over 8 hrs (8 AM to 4 PM) on three consecutive days with concomitant 24 hr urine collections for 17-OHCS and/or UC determinations.

Patients with primary adrenal insufficiency have no rise in the 17-OHCS or UC, whereas patients with secondary adrenal insufficiency will have a subnormal rise on the first day (< 3 times basal 17-OHCS) and will increase to three times the baseline by the third day. A shorter method using a 48 hr continuous infusion (Cortrosyn 0.25 mg in 500 ml normal saline every 12 hrs) is equally valid.

Mineralocorticoids: Excessive mineralocorticoid secretion is suspected in patients with hypertension and hypokalemia. It is important to assess whether the renin-angiotensin system is activated or not. What is the plasma renin activity (PRA)? PRA can be assayed by eliciting a pressure response in an animal (bioassay) but is most often assayed by RIA measuring angiotensin II. Normal values must be established for each method and laboratory. PRA varies with posture, volume status, and sodium content of diet. The PRA is low and the aldosterone production is increased in states of mineralocorticoid excess.

Care must be taken to make sure patients suspected of hyperaldosteronism have volume expansion (Na intake at least 120 meq/day for four days) when measuring urine potassium and aldosterone. Hypokalemia and renal wasting of potassium may resolve with sodium restriction. A urine potassium of > 50 meq/24 hrs is inappropiate in the presence of hypokalemia and suggests aldosterone excess. The normal range for urine aldosterone under sodium loading is < 20 ug/24 hrs. Urine measurements are superior to plasma determinations of aldosterone in making the diagnosis of hyperaldosteronism. However, in differentiating the causes of primary aldosterone excess (adenoma vs hyperplasia), measurement of plasma aldosterone appears to be a better discriminator. Plasma aldosterone, drawn at 8 AM while the patient is recumbent and after being in the supine position overnight, ranges normally between 4 and 12 ng/dl. In patients with an aldosterone-secreting adenoma, plasma levels are > 20 ng/dl. Plasma aldosterone levels in patients with bilateral hyperplasia average 13 ng/dl demonstrating that plasma levels are not helpful in separating these patients from normal subjects.

Adrenal androgens: The adrenal cortex secretes androgens that have weak masculinizing activity. If the concentrations of these weak androgens are high, then some clinical effect is possible (e.g., hirsutism, amenorrhea, voice change, and increased muscle mass in females or prepubertal males). Dehydroepiandrosterone (DHEA) and its conjugated sulfate (DHEA-S) are secreted in milligram amounts each day and are measured as 17-ketosteroids (17-KS) in the urine. Plasma determinations of DHEA-S can be performed on unextracted serum (normal male and female values; 800-3000 ng/ml). Measurement of the serum DHEA-S is often more convenient than collecting 24 hr urine for 17-KS. There are a few occasions when measurement of the serum DHEA-S or urine 17-KS is helpful and these include states of masculinization or virilization.

Adrenal medulla: The catecholamines, norepinephrine and epinephrine, are made in the adrenal medulla. Catecholamines circulate at very low levels in the plasma making determinations of plasma catecholamines technically difficult. However, urine concentration of catecholamines can be readily assayed using fluorometric methods for free norepinephrine (normal, 10 to 70 ug/24 hr) and epinephrine (normal, 0 to 20 ug/24 hr). The metabolites of catecholamines include metanephrine, normetanephrine and vanillylmandelic acid (VMA). Total metanephrines in the urine are < 1.3 mg/24 hrs. Urinary VMA is normally < 7 mg/24 hrs.

Urine studies are ordered when the clinical suspicion for increased adrenergic discharge is high. Are there symptoms that suggest pheochromocytoma (e.g. headache, excessive perspiration, palpitations, hypertension, neuroma, cafe-au-lait spots, multiple endocrine adenomatosis, and family history)? Which study to order is difficult to answer. The biochemical determination one uses is largely dependent on the confidence and the reliability of the laboratory. The VMA performed using the Pisano method is convenient and reliable. Drugs such as thiazide diuretics and the alpha blockers can be used during the urine collection. No special diet is needed while the urine is collected. Any lab that gives normal ranges of VMA up to 10 mg/24 hrs is probably _not_ using this method and those determinations of VMA are less useful in the diagnosis of pheochromocytoma (up to 20 % false negative). Because the free catecholamines are determined by fluorometric assays, many drugs will fluoresce (e.g., tetracyclines, ephredrine nasal spray, alpha-methyldopa) and thus give erroneous values. Urinary total metanephrines are elevated by methyldopa, phenothiazines, and monoamine oxidase inhibitors. Each of the assays (VMA, total metanephrines, free catecholamines) will detect 90 % of the patients with pheochromocytoma. Generally two different studies are helpful in discerning the occasional patient who may have a false negative study. Serial measurements of urines collected daily may smoke out the rare patient with pheochromocytoma that is not seen with one day's collection.

Parathyroid Tests

Serum Calcium: Normal values for total serum calcium vary depending on the laboratory and range between 8.5 and 10.5 mg/dl. About half of the total serum calcium binds to protein (albumin) and the other half circulates as unbound or ionized calcium. Any disturbance in the serum albumin affects the value of the total serum calcium; for each gm of albumin above or below 4 gm/dl changes the serum calcium by about 0.8 mg/dl. For example, a serum calcium of 7.8 mg/dl is normal when the albumin concentration is 3 gm/dl ("corrected" calcium, 8.6 mg/dl). Similarly a serum calcium of 11.0 mg/dl is not abnormal if the serum albumin is 5.0 mg/dl. A serum calcium of 10.5 mg/dl is inappropiately high when the serum albumin is 3.0 gm/dl ("corrected" calcium, 11.5 mg/dl). Many laboratories measure ionized calcium as well as total serum calcium. The parathyroid glands are the primary moment to moment regulators of the serum calcium. The level of ionized calcium determines whether the parathyroid secretes parathyroid hormone (PTH). A low serum ionized calcium stimulates PTH release. PTH causes bone resorption by activating osteoclasts and stimulating osteocytic osteolysis; increases renal hydroxylation of 25-hydroxyvitamin D to form 1,25-dihydroxyvitamin D which stimulates intestinal absorption of calcium; and promotes renal tubular reabsorption of calcium. Each of these actions increases serum calcium which in turn decreases PTH secretion.

Parathyroid Hormone (PTH): Serum PTH levels as assessed by radioimmunoassay (RIA) are one of the least desirable of all RIA assays. There are several reasons: 1) PTH circulates in several heterogeneous states; a result of degradation of the intact (1-84 amino acid) PTH molecule into at least two peptide fragments, the biological inactive C-terminal fragment and the biological active N-terminal fragment (1-34 amino acid). This fragment circulates in much smaller amounts than the C-terminal fragment. 2) Both intact PTH and its fragments are weak antigens. Preparation of antibodies of sufficient specificity and of high titers is difficult since the antigenic response to PTH varies dramatically from animal to animal and from species to species. 3) Most PTH immunoassays cannot distinguish normal levels from low levels of PTH (e.g., PTH levels are "normal" or "low normal" in hypoparathyroidism). If the laboratory has established a reasonably valid assay, then one should interpret PTH values in view of the serum calcium. A "normal" PTH level is inappropriately low for a serum calcium of 6.0 mg/dl and is inappropiately high for a serum calcium of 11.5 mg/dl. Bioassays for PTH such as cytochemical assays are precise and correlate well with clinical states but are time-consuming, technically difficult, and generally unavailable. PTH decreases renal tubular reabsorption of phosphate which leads to phosphaturia and increases renal tubular secretion of cyclic AMP. Phosphate excretion measuring the TmP/GFR is historically one of the oldest methods to assess PTH action. Measurement of urinary cyclic AMP has also been used to assess PTH action.

Nephrogenous cyclic AMP: Urinary cyclic AMP is dependent upon two sources: the filtered load of plasma cyclic AMP and the secretion of cyclic AMP into the urine by the proximal renal tubule (nephrogenous cyclic AMP). This latter component is almost totally dependent on PTH and forms the basis for measuring cyclic AMP excretion. When expressed as a function of the glomerular filtration rate (nanomoles/dl GFR), total urine cyclic AMP is elevated in most patients with hyperparathyroidism. When nephrogenous cyclic AMP is measured, over 90% of patients with hyperparathyroidism have elevated values. Because plasma cyclic AMP measurements are tedious and are necessary for nephrogenous cyclic AMP determination, measurements of nephrogenous cyclic AMP are usually performed in research laboratories. Urine cyclic AMP determinations are helpful in understanding disease states but are rarely helpful clinically. Hypercalcemic patients usually have primary hyperparathyroidism or malignancy. In these situations urinary cyclic AMP lacks specificity for hyperparathyroidism since many patients with tumor-induced hypercalcemia also have increased nephrogenous cyclic AMP values.

References

AvRuskin TW, Tang SC, Juan CS: The glucagon test and growth hormone secretion. J Pediatr 85:102, 1975.

Frohman LA: Diseases of the anterior pituitary, in Felig P, Baxter JD, Broadus AE, Frohman LA (eds): Endocrinology and Metabolism. New York, McGraw-Hill, 1981, pp 151-231.

Health Services Human Growth Hormone Committee: Comparison of the intravenous insulin and oral clonidine tolerance tests for growth hormone secretion. Arch Dis Child 56:852, 1981.

Hershman JM: Use of thyrotropin-releasing hormone in clinical medicine. Med Clin North Am 62:313, 1978.

Liddle GW: Tests of pituitary adrenal suppressibility in the diagnosis of Cushing's syndrome. J Clin Endocrinol Metab 12:1539, 1960.

Rose LI, Williams GH, Lauler DP, Jagger PI: The 48 hour adenocorticotropin infusion test for adrenal insufficiency. Ann Intern Med 73:49, 1970.

Spaulding SW, Utiger RD: The thyroid: physiology, hyperthyroidism, hypothyroidism, and the painful thyroid, in Felig P, Baxter JD, Broadus AE, Frohman LA (eds): Endocrinology and Metabolism. New York, McGraw-Hill, 1981, pp 281-350.

Speckart PF, Nicoloff JT, Bethune JE: Screening for adrenocortical insufficiency with cosyntropin (synthetic ACTH). Arch Intern Med 128:761, 1971.

Spiger M, Jubiz W, Meikle AW, West CD, Tyler FH: Single-dose metyrapone test: review of a four-year experience. Arch Intern Med 135:698, 1975.

Wood JB, James VHT, Frankland AW, Landon J: A rapid test of adrenocortical function. Lancet 1:243, 1965.

Chapter 2

Endocrine Emergencies

DIABETIC KETOACIDOSIS

Diabetic ketoacidosis (DKA) is the most common endocrine emergency. Immediate diagnosis and aggressive management with careful attention to detail can reduce the mortality of this life-threatening disorder to below 2 %. Clinical symptoms of uncontrolled diabetic acidosis include excessive thirst and dry mouth, polyuria, weight loss, air-hunger, nausea (often with vomiting), weakness, muscle aches, headache, abdominal pain, central nervous system depression with drowsiness and stupor which may progress to coma. There are often symptoms related to a coexistent infection. Signs of DKA include: dehydration with dry mucous membranes, dry skin with poor turgor, and sunken eyeballs; tachypnea often deep and labored; a characteristic fruity odor to the breath; tachycardia; and hypotension.

Laboratory evidence of DKA includes: blood glucose is > 300 mg/dl; serum bicarbonate < 15 meq/l; arterial blood pH < 7.30; plasma acetone is positive at 1:2 dilution. The nitroprusside reaction (crushed Acetest tablet on which one drop of diluted plasma is reacted for 2 min) detects acetone and acetoacetate but not beta-hydroxybutyrate, the major ketone body in DKA. Undiluted serum may give a strong acetone reaction in states of starvation alone. The serum potassium may be low, normal, or high but the total body potassium is depleted. The serum sodium is usually normal but may appear low if the serum is lipemic.

Expediency is most important so that one should not wait for every lab result before instituting therapy. Serum electrolytes, plasma glucose, BUN, calcium, phosphorus, magnesium, and CBC are obtained. Urine is collected for analysis and culture if indicated. A bladder catheter is not used in an alert patient. A baseline ECG is obtained and a chest X-ray is usually indicated. Nasogastric suction is necessary for the comatose patient. The management of DKA requires fluid replacement, insulin administration, correction of electrolyte abnormalities, and investigation of precipitating causes. If possible the patient should be treated in an acute care unit where close monitoring is available. Since much of the therapy listed below is administered concommitantly and multiple blood determinations are needed to optimize patient care, a well planned flow sheet (see Appendix, page 152) is a necessity.

Fluid replacement: An intravenous line using at least a 19-gauge needle or catheter is established. The typical adult DKA patient needs 6-10 liters to replete their fluid status. Normal saline is administrated to the hypotensive patient whereas most patients are given 0.45% saline soln (1/2 normal saline) since the plasma osmolality is already greatly elevated. The infusion rate should be rapid (1000 ml for the first 30 min; 1000 ml for next hr; then 300-500 ml/hr over 1st 24 hrs). The rate varies depending on urine output, blood pressure, and the circulatory response to a large volume load. As soon as the blood sugar falls below 250 mg/dl then dextrose 5% (D5/W) is infused.

Insulin administration: There are many regimens for giving regular insulin. Each works as long as there is intensive hourly monitoring of patient's status and recognition of how prior treatment has worked. The use of bolus iv insulin, 2-hourly subcutaneous insulin, hourly intramuscular insulin, or continuous intravenous drip (with or without a starting bolus) doesn't matter; paying close attention to the patient does. Because hypokalemia and hypoglycemia are less frequent with "low dose" regimens, I prefer to give 10 units of regular insulin iv push followed by a constant infusion of 6 U/hr (up to 12 U/hr if there is infection, etc.). If there is no response in the blood sugar or if the acidemia is not being corrected within 3 or 4 hrs, then higher insulin doses are used. Regular insulin is not stopped when the plasma glucose falls below 250 mg/dl but dextrose 5% is started and the amount of insulin infused per hr may be decreased. Intermediate insulin should not be given until the patient is stabilized and able to drink and eat food.

Correct electrolyte abnormalities: Because of the acidemia and osmotic diuresis of DKA a typical patient has lost 600 meq sodium, 400 meq potassium, 400 meq chloride, 400 meq of bicarbonate, and 100 meq of phosphate. If the initial serum K is > 5.5 meq/l, then no KCl is added to the initial iv fluids. If the serum K is normal, then sufficient KCl is added to each liter of fluid so that no more than 40 meq/hr is infused. If the serum K is < 3.5 meq/l, then 40-80 meq/hr are given with close monitoring of ECG and serum K determinations at least every 2 hr. Both the serum K and serum phosphorus fall after fluid and insulin are started and a portion of potassium replacement may be given as potassium phosphate. Any suggestion of renal impairment means less aggressive K replacement.

The serum phosphorus may fall below 1.0 mg/dl during therapy. Phosphate deficiency reduces erythrocyte 2,3-DPG levels increasing hemoglobin affinity for oxygen and decreasing oxygen availabilty to tissue. Although there has been no difference in the mortality or morbidity rates between patients who have had regimens of P replacement and those using standard therapy, phosphorus supplementation has been recommended. Patients with hypophosphatemia on admission are at risk to develop severe hypophosphatemia with insulin therapy and are most likely to benefit from P supplementation. Phosphate may be given at rate of 10-15 mmol/hr in the form of a buffered potassium phosphate solution (Abbott, 3 mmol P/ml and 4 meq K/ml) adding 5 ml of this solution to each liter of intravenous fluid. If P is used, one should measure serum calcium q 4-6 hr since hyperphosphatemia will cause hypocalcemia and possible tetany. Addition of PO4 is contraindicated in renal insufficiency.

The use of bicarbonate therapy in DKA is controversial. There are some good reasons to avoid bicarbonate administration. With acute alkalinization, there is a paradoxical fall of cerebral spinal fluid pH leading to CNS depression (worsening of stupor/coma) and a shift in the hemoglobin oxygen disassociation curve (Bohr effect) leading to tissue hypoxia. However, if the pH is < 7.1 and death is near, then two ampules of sodium bicarbonate (144 meq of Na and HCO3) should be added to a liter of hypotonic saline 0.45% and infused over one hour. Do not give bolus bicarbonate. The goal is to raise the pH to 7.2 - 7.25. Lactate is not used in DKA since some patients, particularly hypotensive subjects, already have elevated blood lactate levels.

Investigate the precipitating cause: This is necessary since any overt or occult infection can lead to DKA. CBC, urine analysis, chest X-ray, and appropiate cultures should be performed as soon as possible. In addition one should consider whether there is an acute myocardial infarction by ECG? Did the diabetic patient take his or her insulin? Was the patient instructed as to what to do in situations where insulin requirements might increase (infection, etc.)? Is the patient hyperthyroid?

Certain risk factors that predispose patients with DKA to higher mortality include: delay in making the diagnosis or instituting appropiate therapy; advanced age; deep coma; uremia; and myocardial infarction. One of the goals of DKA treatment is to educate the patient so that recurrences of DKA can be avoided.

HYPEROSMOLAR COMA

Patients with hyperosmolar nonketotic coma usually have type II diabetes mellitus. They present after an interval (usually 7-14 days) of prolonged osmotic diuresis leading to dehydration. These patients often do not recognize the seriousness of their illness because there is no nausea, vomiting, and air-hunger induced by ketosis. Progressive mental obtundation and convulsions (often focal seizures) lead to medical consultation. The mortality in these patients approaches 40% mainly because of advanced age, complicating illnesses (hypertension, renal insufficiency, congestive heart failure, stroke), and the presentation for medical care late in the illness. There is often some precipitating factor such as pneumonia, sepsis, urinary tract infection, drug administration (diuretics, glucocorticoids, dilantin), intravenous hyperalimentation, tube feeding without sufficient free water, or dialysis.

Laboratory findings include severe hyperglycemia (> 600 mg/dl), hyperosmolality (> 320 mOsm/kg), absent of ketosis, and azotemia (BUN 60-90 mg/dl). The plasma osmolality is calculated using the following formula: 2 (Na + K) + glucose/18 + BUN/2.8 . The serum sodium may be low as a result of the prolonged hyperglycemia. The correction factor is 1.6 meq/l of Na for each 100 mg glucose/dl above normal serum glucose levels. Patients with normal or elevated serum sodium still have total body depletion of sodium as well as K, Mg, and P. If the bicarbonate is low (< 15 meq/l) in the absent of ketonemia, one should think of lactic acidosis.

The treatment is similar to that for DKA. These patients need large amount of fluids (up to 10 l) given as normal saline. Monitoring of central venous pressure or pulmonary wedge pressure is often necessary to aid in the management of fluids in patients with renal and cardiac failure. As in DKA meticulous attention to input and output, measurement of serum electrolytes, insulin therapy, an up-to-date flow sheet, and idenitification of precipitating events are important.

HYPOGLYCEMIC COMA

Severe hypoglycemia is a medical emergency and causes mental confusion, bizarre behavoir, seizures, coma, and finally death. Hypoglycemia should be considered in any comatose patient in whom a specific diagnosis is not established. Insulin-induced hypoglycemia ("insulin reaction"), a complication of insulin therapy for diabetes mellitus, accounts for the majority of the cases of hypoglycemia. Management of hypoglycemic coma requires urgency to prevent brain damage:

1) Obtain blood for plasma glucose determination. Plasma can be stored for insulin measurement if the cause of hypoglycemia is not known.

2) Administer 50 ml of 50% dextrose intravenously over a 3-5 min period. If the patient does not awake during this interval, administer another 50 ml of 50% dextrose. If the patient recovers after dextrose, start dextrose 5% in water until hourly blood sugars reveal no hypoglycemia. If oral agents have been ingested, the follow-up interval relates to the type of agent and its biological half-life and may be prolonged (e.g., the effects of chlorpropamide may last up to 60 hrs).

3) Investigate the precipitating factors (see Hypoglycemia, page 53).

Remember glucose administration for alcohol-induced hypoglycemia can unmask thiamine deficiency producing Wernicke's disease (weakness and paralysis of external ocular recti, nystagmus, various palsies of conjugate gaze; ataxia; deranged mental function).

ACUTE ADRENAL INSUFFICIENCY

Adrenal crisis is relatively easy to manage; the difficult aspect is to think of the possibility of adrenal insufficiency. The symptoms are nonspecific (weakness and fatigue, weight loss, anorexia). Patients with undiagnosed Addison's disease may present with nausea, vomiting, fever, hypotension and vascular collapse precipitated by a variety of stresses including infection, trauma, surgery, drugs, cathartics, enemas, and fasting.

One clinical finding suggesting Addison's disease is cutaneous hyperpigmentation particularly in the creases of hand, over the knuckles, in the axilla, on the gingival mucosa, in the areola of the breasts, and in the perineum. Scars formed after adrenal insufficiency develops may be pigmented. Vitiligo is also a clue signaling an autoimmune disorder--the most common cause of adrenal insufficiency.

Patients with pituitary disease are also at risk to develop secondary adrenal insufficiency, but the hyperpigmentation typical of Addison's disease will be absent. Bilateral adrenal hemorrhage leading to crisis (hypotension, fever, nausea and vomiting, confusion) is a rare occurrence and usually found in patients with complicated medical illnesses especially those on anticoagulants. They manifest crisis symptoms in addition to abdominal, flank, or back pain. Hyperpigmentation and weight loss are absent.

Common laboratory findings in adrenal crisis include hyponatremia, hyperkalemia and azotemia; anemia, eosinophilia, lymphocytosis, hypoglycemia, and hypercalcemia are less frequent. Plasma cortisol is low.

The management of adrenal crisis requires prompt clinical diagnosis, taking of blood for cortisol and ACTH determinations, replacement of fluids to combat dehydration and shock, cortisol administration, and identification and treatment of any precipitating causes. Once the diagnosis is suspected, blood is drawn for plasma cortisol and ACTH determination and therapy is begun at once. This is an emergency situation and treatment is life-saving:

A large intravenous line is used to give one to two liters of normal saline-dextrose 5% over the first two hrs. Hydrocortisone sodium succinate (Solu-Cortef) 100 mg is given iv stat, and 100 mg q 6 hr is administered as continuous iv drip over the first 24 hrs. Solu-Cortef is reduced to 50 mg iv q 6 hr when conditions stabilize. Mineralocorticoids are not needed since cortisol at these large doses (> 150 mg/day) has enough salt retaining activity. Three to five liters of saline are given during the first 24 hrs.

If the previously drawn plasma cortisol returns low and ACTH levels are available, the work-up is considerably simplified since a low cortisol value and elevated ACTH confirm the diagnosis of Addison's disease. If ACTH levels are not available, then a Cortrosyn study (see page 16-18) should be done after the crisis is passed. A confirmed diagnosis means a need for chronic maintenance therapy, for education as to what to do in stress situations, and for wearing an identification medallion (Medic-Alert) stating the medical diagnosis.

MYXEDEMA COMA

The diagnosis of myxedema coma should be considered in every case of stupor or coma state with hypothermia and in which there is no other obvious cause. (Hypoglycemia is another endocrine disorder presenting in a similar manner). Myxedema coma is the rare and very serious (mortality up to 66%) end stage of hypothyroidism. Most often the patient has had unrecognized hypothyroidism for some time where a precipitating event leads to myxedema coma. Precipitating factors include pulmonary infection, congestive heart failure, general anesthesia and surgery, drugs (sedatives, narcotics, antidepressants), and exposure to cold. An elderly person not known to have hypothyroidism may develop myxedema coma during the winter; a history of previous thyroid hormone therapy, of radioactive iodine treatment; a thyroidectomy scar; or goiter are clues to the correct diagnosis. In addition, the patient usually has physical findings of prolonged hypothyroidism (dry skin, puffy eyelids and face, large tongue, hyporeflexia, bradycardia).

Respiratory failure is the major cause of death in myxedema coma. The respiratory center becomes insensitive to hypercarbia and hypoxia creating vicious cycle of progressive respiratory depression, reduced cardiac output and increasing cerebral hypoxia. Pulmonary infection often complicates these events. Hypoventilation leads to hypercapnia and respiratory acidosis. Hypotension and hypothermia are present. Additional findings include dilutional hyponatremia, anemia, and occasionally hypoglycemia and cortisol deficiency. Blood should be drawn for laboratory testing (T4-RIA, T3U, TSH, plasma cortisol), but treatment should not be delayed awaiting the thyroid results.

Myxedema coma should be treated in an acute care unit since these patients often require ventilatory assistance. Drugs that suppress respiration should be avoided and any infection treated vigorously. Hypothermia should be corrected by passive warming with blankets and rather than active warming devices which increase caloric need, induce peripheral vasodilation, and accentuate the hypotension.

Thyroid hormone replacement is essential and most endocrinologists use large doses of L-thyroxine (T4) iv. This is a paradox compared to the usual treatment of hypothyroidism where small doses of thyroxine are titrated over several weeks to euthyroid state. The potential risk of aggressive therapy is accepted in view of the mortality rate in myxedema coma. Thyroxine 500 ug is given as iv bolus. This dose saturates thyroxine binding sites which serve as a depot for free T4. I also recommend glucocorticoid coverage (Solu-Cortef 100 mg q 6 hr iv drip) until results of the initial plasma cortisol is known. Temperature, pulse, blood pressure and mental status should improve within 24 hrs. Intravenous fluids should be administrated carefully. Hyponatremia will be corrected by thyroxine alone; no saline administration is necessary. A maintenance dose of T4 50-100 ug as a single daily bolus iv is given until oral medications can be taken. At that time L-thyroxine 2 ug/kg body wt/day po is prescribed.

THYROID CRISIS

Thyroid crisis ("thyroid storm") is a clinical diagnosis that is difficult to discern from severe thyrotoxicosis since the serum thyroxine and serum triiodothyronine levels are identical. Thyroid crisis almost always develops in an undiagnosed hyperthyroid patient who has a major stress precipitating the following clinical syndrome: a severely ill subject with fever (> 100° F), marked anxiety and agitation, anorexia with nausea and vomiting, tachycardia (tachydysrhythmias), abdominal pain, pulmonary edema, or cardiac failure. These occur in the setting of other symptoms and signs of hyperthyroidism. Elderly patients may not demonstrate agitation or goiter but rather show apathy, confusion, cachexia and atrial fibrillation. The precipitating stress may be a medical illness (infection, DKA, etc.) or a surgical procedure or trauma (e.g., hip fracture). Thyroid storm used to be a major problem during surgery for toxic goiter, but proper treatment making the patient euthyroid prior to surgery has alleviated this concern.

The treatment of thyroid crisis requires vigorous management of underlying illness; supportive measures to decrease body temperature; beta-adrenergic blockade of the catechol-mimetic signs and symptoms of thyrotoxicosis; inhibition of thyroid hormone synthesis; blockade of thyroid hormone release from the thyroid gland; and inhibition of the conversion of T4 to T3. Supportive measures include digoxin for heart failure (the usual dose needs to be increased 1.5-2 fold), antipyretics (acetaminophen or corticosteroids but not aspirin since it displaces thyroid hormones from their binding proteins), a cooling blanket for high fever, and iv fluids supplemented with B vitamins. In the nauseated patient propranolol 1 mg should be given as iv boluses every 10-15 min (no more than 15-20 mg should be given iv). Later propranolol can be given po 160-320 mg/day. The major effect is beta-adrenergic blockade but propranolol also diminishes the peripheral conversion of T4 to T3. Propylthiouracil (PTU) 1000 mg should be given po or be crushed given via nasogastric tube; thereafter 300 mg PTU is given q 4-6 hrs. It takes 10-20 days to reach maximum PTU effect, but the thionamides (PTU and methimazole) are the mainstay therapy for hyperthyroidism. PTU also blocks T4 to T3 conversion. One hour after the loading dose of PTU is given, sodium iodide 1 gm is given iv drip over 12 hrs q 12 hr to block preformed thyroid hormone release from the thyroid gland. If iodine is given prior to PTU, it may fuel the synthesis of more T4 possibly worsening the clinical state. Iodine is the most effective agent for lowering serum thyroxine acutely. If the patient can tolerate po meds, then Lugol's solution 10 gtt q 8 hr or saturated solution of potassium iodide (SSKI) 5 gtt q 8 hr will serve as well as sodium iodide iv. The effect of iodine may last only a few weeks, but by then the thionamides should reach peak efficacy. Although there is no evidence of adrenal insufficiency in thyroid storm, high dose glucocorticoids do block the conversion of T4 to T3 and lower body temperature. Thus dexamethasone 2 mg iv q 6 hr is recommended for 24-48 hrs.

In the treatment of thyroid crisis the patient should improve markedly during the first 12 hrs even before serum T4 falls. The patient's temperature, tachycardia, tremor, and mental status will improve during the first day's treatment, but the congestive heart failure may take days to resolve, and the atrial fibrillation up to two weeks to revert to normal rhythmn. Muscle weakness may improve during the first few hours after therapy, but strength returns to normal only weeks later.

HYPERCALCEMIC CRISIS

The signs and symptoms of severe hypercalcemia are not specific. The patient may have hyperparathyroidism or some other medical illness frequently associated with hypercalcemia (e.g., malignancy). In this setting, an intercurrent disorder such as a viral infection or progression of the underlying disease leads to anorexia, nausea, vomiting, and weakness. The combination of inadequate fluid intake and the inability of hypercalcemic patients to conserve free water leads to volume contraction which raise the total serum calcium level to over 14-15 mg/dl. The degree of calcemia needs to be interpreted in relation to the serum protein concentration since approximately 1/2 of the serum calcium is bound to albumin; the other 1/2 (ionized or free Ca) is the metabolically active component. In general, for each gm/dl of albumin above or below 4 gm/dl, the serum calcium can be "adjusted" upwards or downwards by 0.8 mg/dl. For example if the serum calcium is 12 mg/dl and the albumin 2 gm/dl, then the "corrected" serum is nearly 14 gm/dl which has much more significance. The magnitude of the hypercalcemia correlates well with the severity of the clinical status. Dehydration, confusion, and lethargy are signs that should trigger aggressive management. Untreated severe hypercalcemia leads to coma, muscular paralysis, and ventricular arrhythmia (QT shortening on the ECG).

Management of hypercalcemic crisis involves volume repletion and hydration. A large bore indwelling intravenous needle is used to deliver 1000 ml of normal saline during the 1st hr realizing that these patients are at least 4-5 l deficient in fluid. Thereafter normal saline is infused at 250-300 ml/hr. Volume repletion will often decrease the hypercalcemia to less than critical levels (< 13 mg/dl).

If the clinical status is not satisfactory after hydration alone, then the renal excretion of calcium can be enhanced by saline diuresis. The rate of saline administration must be individualized depending on cardiac and renal status. Central venous pressure monitoring is helpful. After hydration is assured, furosemide 40-60 mg q 4-6 hr is given iv with careful recording of input and output. Urine volumes losses are replaced with intravenous normal saline. With these measures the serum calcium will generally fall 3-4 mg/dl within 24 hrs. If renal function will not permit saline diuresis, peritoneal or hemodialysis can reduce the calcium concentration.

Another effective means to lower serum calcium is to decrease bone resorption. Since increased resorption of bone is the etiology of 99% of hypercalcemias, any agent that blocks osteoclastic function will lower the serum calcium. Mithramycin is the most effective agent. At a concentration 1/10 of its therapeutic dose in treating testicular neoplasm, mithramycin inhibits osteoclast differentiation. Within 24-48 hrs after mithramycin (25 ug/kg iv over 8 hrs) the serum calcium will fall and stay reduced for 7-14 days. If no effect is seen within 24 hrs, another course is used. The major side effect is thrombocytopenia which occurs infrequently.

Calcitonin also decreases serum calcium but not as well or for as long as mithramycin. The potential side effects of calcitonin are small compared to mitramycin. Salmon calcitonin, 2-8 MRC units/kg, is given sc q 12 hrs. The hypocalcemic effect lasts for 48-72 hr after which tachyphylaxis usually develops.

Medications that sometimes lower serum calcium include the following: Glucocorticoids (prednisone 40-60 mg/day) decrease the serum calcium in some malignancies, in sarcoidosis, and in vitamin A and D intoxication. Salicylates (600 mg q 6 hr) or indomethacin (75-150 mg/day) inhibit prostanglandin synthetase which might cause the humoral hypercalcemia of malignancy, but their efficiency is sporadic and unpredictable. Intravenous phosphates work well, but the precipitation of Ca-PO4 salts within body tissues has lead to very infrequent use. If malignant disease is susceptible to chemotherapy, then these agents should be used.

Since immobilization tends to exacerbate hypercalcemia, early ambulation is strongly recommended. Oral phosphates (10 ml phosphosoda tid) may be used in some chronic hypercalcemic patients particularly if renal function is normal.

If primary hyperparathyroidism was the cause of the hypercalcemic crisis, then surgical intervention is recommended.

HYPOCALCEMIC CRISIS

Hypocalcemia causes neuromuscular irritability. The severity of neurologic disorder correlates with the degree of hypocalcemia. It is the ionized calcium level which is the crucial factor rather than the total serum calcium. In the absence of any serum protein abnormalities or any acid-base derangements, the total serum calcium is quite reliable in assessing the calcemic status. Acute hyperventilation is a condition in which the total serum calcium is normal but the ionized calcium is low due to increased protein binding of calcium in alkaline conditions. Hypoalbuminemia of chronic disease leads to hypocalcemia but not to any clinical hypocalcemic syndrome since the ionized calcium is normal. Acidosis raises serum ionized calcium levels.

Hypocalcemic crisis presents as overt tetany: carpopedal spasm, spasm of the laryngeal muscles with stridor, muscle cramps, and occasionally as a seizure. Chronic hypocalcemia sometimes presents with papilledema related to benign intracranial hypertension. Cardiac arrhythmias are seen with the typical ECG finding of a prolonged QT interval caused by ST lengthening. The cause of the hypocalcemia may be obvious: operative parathyroid damage related to thyroid or parathyroid surgery; multiple blood transfusions (citrate complexes calcium and, if not metabolized by the liver, leads to hypocalcemia); acute pancreatitis; or rickets and osteomalacia. Hypocalcemia due to idiopathic hypoparathyroidism, vitamin D deficiency (e.g., gastrointestinal disease with malabsorption), or hypomagnesemia may not be so obvious. Hypomagnesemic hypocalcemia is frequent in chronic alcoholics and is occasionally found in patients with intestinal malabsorption syndromes. Whenever the total body's Mg is low (serum Mg < 1.2 mg/dl), PTH synthesis and release is inhibited leading to hypocalcemia. Correction of the hypomagnesemia restores normocalcemia.

Hypocalcemic tetany must be distinguished from the muscle spasms that result from Clostridium tetanii infection of a wound. The spasms of tetanus begin in the head and neck (trismus) whereas the spasms of tetany occur in the extremities (carpopedal spasm). Strychnine poisoning presents with clonic spasms not tetanic spasms. Seizures in infants caused by hypocalcemia may be aggravated by usual treatment with anticonvulsants since dilantin and phenobarbital decrease vitamin D levels and leads to less calcium absorption by the intestine.

Emergency laboratory assessment requires immediate serum calcium and ECG to assess the QT interval. Serum for magnesium, phosphorus, total protein/albumin, BUN, electrolytes, and PTH levels are obtained prior to therapy.

Hypocalcemic crisis is treated iv infusion calcium of 10-20 ml of 10% calcium gluconate (90-180 mg of elemental calcium) over 10 min to immediately ameliorate the signs and symptoms of hypocalcemia. Concentrated calcium is very irritating to the veins so dilution of 2 ten ml ampules of calcium gluconate into 100 ml of 5% dextrose infused over 10-15 min is preferable. This may be repeated every 4-6 hrs for recurrence of symptoms. Although the serum calcium falls quickly to pretreatment levels after the iv bolus, hypocalcemic symptoms and signs may not return for several hours. Alternatively a constant infusion of 15 mg calcium/kg every 4-6 hr may be given. Calcium gluconate 10% has 9 mg of elemental calcium/ml of solution. Monitoring of serum calcium level is important. If hypomagnesemia is found, then magnesium sulfate 1 gm (8.13 meq or 98 mg of elemental Mg) given im tid for 3-5 days will replace body reserves and correct the hypocalcemia. For patient taking iv fluids an intravenous drip of MgSO4 (98-196 mg q 8 hrs for 3-5 days) can be used to avoid painful im injections. For transfusion hypocalcemia, 10 ml of 10% calcium chloride should be given for every two units of citrated blood. Finally those patients with chronic hypocalcemia (page 123) who require calcium supplementation and vitamin D replacement need to wear proper identification as to their medical diagnosis (e.g., Medic-Alert).

Patients who have diabetes mellitus, diabetes insipidus, adrenal insufficiency, hypoparathyroidism, and those receiving chronic glucocorticoids should carry a card or preferably a bracelet or medallion listing diagnosis, medications, and attending physician. The lack of such information could prove diastrous in emergency situations when the patient is not conscious. Bracelets and medallions are available from the following non-profit organization:

Medic-Alert Foundation International
1000 North Palm Street
P.O. Box 1009
Turlock, CA 95380

References

Arieff AL, Carrol JH: Non-ketotic hyperosmolar coma with hyperglycemia: clinical features, pathophysiology, renal function, acid-base balance, plasma-cerebral fluid equilibria, and the effects of therapy. Medicine 51:73, 1972.

Braverman LE: Thyroid Storm, in Krieger DT, Bardin CW (eds): Current Therapy in Endocrinology 1983-1984. Burlington, Ontario, BC Decker, 1983, pp 65-69.

Fisher JN, Shahshahani MN, Kitabchi AE: Diabetic ketoacidosis: low dose insulin therapy by various routes. N Engl J Med 297:238, 1977.

Foster DW: Insulin deficiency and hyperosmolar coma. Adv Intern Med 19:159, 1974.

Foster DW, McGarry JD: The metabolic derangements and treatment of diabetic ketoacidosis. N Engl J Med 309:159, 1983.

Holvey DN, Goodner CJ, Nicoloff JT, Dawbrig JT: Treatment of myxedema coma with intravenous thyroxine. Arch Intern Med 113:89, 1964.

McKenna TJ: Acute adrenal insufficiency. Hosp Med 12:77, 1976.

Rapoport B: Myxedema coma, in Krieger DT, Bardin CW (eds): Current Therapy in Endocrinology 1983-1984. Burlington, Ontario, BC Decker, 1983, pp 75-80.

Schade DS, Eaton RP, Alberti KGMM, Johnston DG: Diabetic Coma: Ketoacidotic and Hyperosmolar. Albuquerque, Univ of New Mexico Press, 1981.

Schneider AB, Sherwood LM: Pathogenesis and management of hypoparathyroidism and other hypocalcemic disorders. Metabolism 24:871, 1975.

Suki WN, Yium JJ, Von Minden M, Saller-Hebert C, Eknoyan G, Martinez-Maldonado M: Acute treatment of hypercalcemia with furosemide. N Engl J Med 283:836, 1970.

Chapter 3

Diabetes Mellitus

Diabetes mellitus is the most common endocrine disorder encountered in medical practice. The complications of this chronic disorder of glucose homeostasis are a major cause of disability and morbidity.

DIAGNOSIS:

Diabetes mellitus is easily diagnosed when there is unequivocal elevation of the plasma glucose (> 200 mg/dl) with classical symptoms of polyuria, polydipsia, polyphagia, and weight loss. Some patients may not have this degree of hyperglycemia or these symptoms. In these patients an oral glucose tolerance test (GTT) is used to establish the diagnosis of diabetes mellitus. The National Diabetes Study Group has made recommendations for the standardization of testing and has established criteria for the diagnosis of diabetes mellitus which are very useful. By these criteria, diabetes mellitus is present when:

1) Fasting plasma glucose $\geq$ 140 mg/dl on two occasions or
2) Fasting plasma glucose < 140 mg/dl and 2 hr plasma glucose $\geq$ 200 mg/dl with one intervening value > 200 mg/dl following a 75 gm glucose load (GTT).

Normal glucose values of non-pregnant adults are: fasting plasma glucose < 115 mg/dl; 2 hr plasma glucose < 140 mg/dl. Remember: older tests give criteria for whole blood but most glucose determinations are now performed on plasma with results that average 15% higher than whole blood glucose.

Glucose tolerance testing is not recommended in the following circumstances:

1) when fasting hyperglycemia is already present,
2) in hospitalized patients or acutely ill patients or patients who are physically inactive (e.g., bedridden), or
3) subjects taking medications such as diuretics, propranolol, dilantin, glucocorticoids, estrogens, and birth control pills.

The GTT should be performed only on subjects who have been on an unrestricted diet containing at least 300 gm of carbohydrate/day and who have been physically active for 3 days prior to the test. A 75 gm glucose load should be administrated in the morning after a 10 hr fast. The patient should remained seated and should not smoke during the study. Blood is drawned at 0, 30, 60, 90, and 120 min.

Some patients have impaired glucose tolerance (fasting plasma glucose < 140 mg/dl; 2 hr plasma glucose > 140 mg/dl; and an intervening value > 200 mg/dl) following the 75 gm load. These subjects have an abnormality in glucose metabolism intermediate between normal and overt diabetes. It may worsen to diabetes, improve toward normal, or remain unchanged on serial testing. It is best to label these patients as having impaired glucose tolerance and not diabetes mellitus.

Glucose tolerance tests on pregnant women are interpreted somewhat differently. The criteria for gestational diabetes mellitus are those of O'Sullivan. Diabetes mellitus is diagnosed during GTT when two or more plasma glucose concentrations which meet or exceed the following criteria: fasting plasma glucose 105 mg/dl; 1 hr, 190 mg/dl; 2 hr, 165 mg/dl; 3 hr, 145 mg/dl. Pregnant females normally have fasting glucoses 10-30 mg/dl below the subject's non-pregnant fasting value.

CLASSIFICATION:

Diabetes mellitus Type I: Patients who are insulin deficient due to islet cell loss are dependent upon replacement therapy. Type I diabetes mellitus usually has its onset in youth. These patients are prone to ketosis and often present in diabetic ketoacidosis. Type I diabetes is frequently associated with specific HLA types which may predispose to viral insulitis or autoimmune phenomena (e.g., islet cell antibodies). The inheritance is complex and not simple Mendelian inheritance. The family history is as likely to be negative as positive for diabetes mellitus Type I. Even if an identical twin develops Type I diabetes mellitus, the other twin has only a 50% chance of developing diabetes.

Diabetes mellitus Type II: This is the common form of diabetes, seen typically in overweight adults. At least 80% of these patients are obese. The hyperglycemia is secondary to tissue insensitivity to circulating insulin (insulin resistance). The plasma levels of insulin are often elevated but less than one would expect in normal subjects given the same degree of hyperglycemia, and there is a delay in insulin secretion following glucose challenge. The family history is usually positive and often shows the pattern of autosomal dominant inheritance. Type II patients are resistant to the development of ketosis since they have enough insulin to inhibit lipolysis. A small subset of Type II patients develop diabetes at an early age (maturity-onset diabetes of youth or MODY).

Secondary Diabetes Mellitus: This form of diabetes results from loss of pancreatic tissue due to pancreatitis or surgery, or from hormonal antagonism to insulin action as in acromegaly and Cushing's syndrome.

Impaired Glucose Tolerance designates glucose tolerance results intermediate between normal and overt diabetes. This has been discussed in relation to the GTT. The basis of this separate classification rather than including it in Type II diabetes is the observation that the development of overt diabetes in such patients occurs normally at a rate of 1-5 %/year. Such an impairment of glucose tolerance may not be associated with long-term microangiopathic and neuropathic complications of diabetes mellitus.

Lipotrophic Diabetes Mellitus is a rare hyperglycemic syndrome characterized by severe insulin resistance, partial or total absence of body fat, high circulating levels of insulin, absence of ketosis, and hepatomegaly which often progresses to cirrhosis.

COMPLICATIONS:

The long-term complications of diabetes mellitus are the same regardless of the classification of diabetes (Type I, Type II, or secondary diabetes). Chronic hyperglycemia leads to hyperlipidemia, hypercholesterolemia, and glycosylation of proteins that are presumed to cause microvascular and atherosclerotic changes.

Diabetic Retinopathy: Background (non-proliferative retinopathy) is characterized histologically by outpouchings of capillary walls (microaneurysms) and clinically by "dot" or "blot" hemorrhages, soft gray-white exudates (representing microinfarction of superficial nerve fibers), and retinal edema. Although microaneurysms can not be seen with the ophthalmoscope, intra-retinal hemorrhages or (dot or blot hemorrhages) can be detected with the ophthalmoscope. Background retinopathy increases with the duration of the disease such that half of the patients with diabetes mellitus for 10 yrs will manifest this form of retinopathy. It usually does not cause any visual impairment unless retinal edema, plaques of hard exudates, or hemorrhage occur in the macula itself.

Proliferative retinopathy is an entirely different story. Diabetes is the leading cause of blindness in the United States mainly due to proliferative retinopathy. New vessels, containing no mural pericytes to support their endothelium, are very fragile. These new vessels proliferate in response to ischemia and are most often seen at the disc margin. Because of their fragility these vessels are subject to hemorrhage into the retina and vitreous. The finding of proliferative retinopathy has significant clinical importance. The incidence of severe visual loss increases from 1.5%/yr to nearly 20%/yr after proliferative retinopathy is first identified. Fluorescein angiography is helpful in evaluating retinopathy since it identifies severe intra-retinal hemorrhage and early neovascularization. Treatment consists of photocoagulation to decrease oxygen requirements throughout the retina and thus retard the neovascular process. In cases of persistent vitreous hemorrhage which have not cleared over a year, surgical removal of the vitreous (vitrectomy) has been relatively successful in restoring useful vision.

Diabetic Nephropathy: Urinary tract infections are common in diabetics and need to be treated appropriately. Microvascular changes in the kidney, including thickening of the basement membrane and mesangium of the glomerulus, are associated with increased glomerular permeability resulting in proteinuria. Proteinuria of 3-5 gms/day can result in hypoalbuminemia and edema (nephrotic syndrome). Persistent proteinuria is an ominous sign since renal failure usually develops within five years after its appearance. Once azotemia is present, progressive development to frank uremia occurs within 3-4 years on the average. Hypertension most often follows renal insufficiency and is found in over 70% of patients with diabetic nephropathy. Treatment of diabetic renal failure is difficult. The criteria for institution of hemodialysis or renal transplantation have to be formulated in view of each center's experience since these patients do not fare as well as those with non-diabetic renal failure.

Diabetic Neuropathy: Diabetic neuropathy is one of the earliest clinically detectable complications of diabetes mellitus. Of the several forms of diabetic neuropathy, peripheral neuropathy (symmetrical segmental demyelination of long nerve axons) is most common and is manifest by loss of ankle jerks and decreased vibratory sensation. Patients complain of an insidious onset of numbness, tingling, and a burning sensation which is characteristically worse at night. Ultimately there is a glove-and-stocking loss of pin prick and light touch sensation. Neurotrophic ulcers may develop in areas of repeated trauma (such as that due to poorly fitted shoes or to unattended callus). The loss of pain perception may lead to neurotropic arthropathy (Charcot joints) which are typically located in the tarsal-metatarsal area bilaterally.

Mononeuropathy is a disorder of a single nerve or nerve root (typically the femoral, sciatic, lateral femoral cutaneous, or the third cranial nerves) thought to be due to infarction following occlusion of a vasa nervorum. Pain in the distribution of the affected nerve is the most troublesome symptom. The diabetic third nerve palsy (ptosis, ophthalmoplegia) can be differentiated from a more ominous intracranial process (aneurysm, caverous sinus thrombosis) by preservation of the pupillary response to light in the diabetic-related mononeuropathy. Mono-neuropathy usually has a good prognosis with spontaneous return of function and resolution of pain within 3-18 months.

Diabetic amyotrophy leads to weakness of the pelvic girdle muscles, or less commonly, the shoulder muscles. There is no associated pain. Diabetic amyotrophy is best seen in the hands with wasting of the interosseous muscles particularly over the dorsum next to the 2nd metacarpal bone (1st dorsal interosseous muscle).

Autonomic neuropathy produces postural hypotension, impotence, retrograde ejaculation, hypotonic bladder, gastroparesis, and diabetic diarrhea.

Management of the polyneuropathy is directed to symptomatic relief of pain with non-narcotic analgesics, exquisite foot care (toe nails trimmed, avoidance of hot water soaks, proper fitting shoes, gentle abrasion of corns and calluses with a pumice stone). Better control of the diabetes may improve the neurological symptoms. Treatment with medications is still very empirical; a variety have been tried and each regimen has had its proponents. Such medications include amitriptyline (50-100 mg hs often prescribed with fluphenazine 1 mg, if no effect in six weeks then discontinue), dilantin (100 mg tid, discontinue in two weeks if there is no effect), carbamazepine (starting with 200 mg/day increasing up to 800 mg/day, if no effect at this dose then discontinue), antihistamines (diphenhydramine 50 mg tid), and vitamin preparations such as Brewer's yeast tablets (three tabs qid). All have met with varying success.

Atherosclerotic Cardiovascular Disease: Arteriosclerosis is accelerated in diabetes mellitus; as a result, coronary artery disease and peripheral vascular disease are significant causes of morbidity and mortality. The post-mortum incidence of coronary artery occlusion is 5 times more frequent in diabetics than in the non-diabetics in all decades of life and regardless of sex. The immediate mortality rate of acute myocardial infarction is similar to the non-diabetic population (30-55%), but the long term prognosis in the diabetic is quite different with a five year survival of 38-43% compared to 49-83% in non-diabetics. Diabetic females are as likely to have myocardial infarction as diabetic males.

Peripheral artery occlusion is a common complication leading to claudication, rest pain, ulcer formation, and gangrene. Peripheral arterial disease is often associated with diabetic neuropathy and local infection, leading to the "diabetic foot." Five out of every six major leg amputations for ischemic disease of the foot occur in patients with diabetes mellitus. As a general rule, arteriosclerosis in diabetes mellitus has an increased incidence, occurs at an earlier age, is more rapidly progressive and accentuated, and carries a more severe prognosis than in non-diabetics.

MANAGEMENT:

Probably nowhere else in medical therapeutics are there more ways to manage a problem than in diabetes mellitus. The ideal management of diabetes would lead to a normal life style; normal glucose, fat, and protein metabolism; avoidance of hypoglycemia; prevention of long-term complications; and satisfactory psychosocial adaptation to living with a chronic disease. These goals can be achieved in acute diabetes (diabetic ketoacidosis, hyperosmolar coma), but are usually only transiently achieved in the day-to-day care of patients with diabetes mellitus. Sixty years of experience with insulin therapy have not prevented the long-term complications of this disorder. There are abundant laboratory data to suggest that achievement of euglycemia is the best way to prevent these complications. Although 20% of patients with diabetes mellitus never develop complications, there is no way to detect these "protected" patients in advance. The author believes that the best method to avoid long-term complications of diabetes is to maintain the blood sugar as close to normal as possible. If the physician's attitude is lackadaisical, this philosophy is transferred to the patient and reflects how he or she will handle his or her diabetes.

The most crucial time to share the philosophy of management as well as the specifics on how to achieve these goals is immediately after the diagnosis is made (1st office visit, 1st hospitalization). It is very difficult to change

life habits once they are established. The time to initiate
regular diet, weight control, insulin dosage, etc. is not
when the patient finally presents with symptomatic
neuropathy, claudication, or loss of vision. To prevent
these complications requires a committed approach early in
the disease. Patient education is the primary factor in
achieving adequate control. A team approach which uses the
expertise of a dietician, diabetic teaching nurse, and
physician is ideal. A check list (see Appendix, page
153-154) helps to insure that the patient receives optimal
instructions.

Diet and Weight Control: A well-balanced diet eaten
regularly at breakfast, lunch, and dinner (bedtime snack for
those patients receiving insulin) is necessary. A diet
composed of 50% carbohydrate, 20% protein, and 30% fat is
reasonable but food preferences and socio-economic
situations should be used to determine the precise regimen.
Consultation with the dietician is quite helpful.

The number of Calories (kcal) recommended is based on
body weight and activity. Ideal body weight (IBW) for adult
females with a medium frame approximates 100 lbs plus 5 lbs
for each inch over 5 ft. Thus, a 5'2" women's IBW is 110
lbs. For a small frame, deduct 10% from IBW; for large
frame, add 10% of IBW. For medium frame males the IBW is
106 lbs plus 5 lbs/in over 5 ft. Deduct or add 10% of IBW
if small or large frame respectively. Thus, a 6'1" large
frame man's IBW would be 188 lbs [106 + (5 x 13)] + 10% [106
+ (5 x 13)].

The total calorie requirement each day is the sum of the
basal requirements plus the activity requirements. Basal
calorie requirement is figured as IBW times a factor of 10
(IBW x 10). The calorie requirement based on activity for a
sedentary life style is IBW x 3; moderate activity, IBW x 5;
and heavy work, IBW x 10. Thus, a 5'10" medium frame
construction worker would require 1560 Calories (IBW x 10)
plus 1560 Calories (assume heavy worker-156 x 10) for a
total of 3120 Calories each day to maintain body weight.

When patients need weight reduction decreasing total
calorie intake to 500 Calories/day less than maintenance
will produce a 1 lb weight loss each week (-1000
Calories/day will give a 2 lb weight reduction each week).
All patients need repeated dietary instructions to reinforce
dietary habits.

Insulin Treatment: The Type I diabetic patient will
require insulin to lower blood glucose. If there is some
"reserve" of insulin secretory activity from the pancreatic
beta cell, then blood sugar is more easily regulated. The

amount and type of insulin required will vary and is dependent on dietary intake, activity, and whether there is any residual endogenous insulin production.

Patients with Type I diabetes are generally started on an intermediate-acting insulin (NPH, Lente, or Monotard). This may be done as an outpatient when the patient has only modest symptoms but many patients will already be hospitalized after presenting with ketoacidosis (see DKA page 23). To start 15-25 units (U) of NPH or Lente insulin are given sc 30-60 min prior to breakfast. Patients are an active participant in the care of their diabetes. They are responsible for insulin injections and for testing and recording their blood glucose or urine sugar before meals and bedtime. Monitoring these variables is the only way to assess whether the insulin regimen is controlling the diabetes. Control is difficult to define. The level of hyperglycemia must be arbitrarily set for each patient and their particular circumstance. For example, the degree of hyperglycemia permitted may be greater for a 75 yr old subject than for an otherwise healthy 23 yr old individual mainly because of the risks of hypoglycemia (insulin reaction) in the elderly. In general, a preprandial blood glucose of < 150 mg/dl represents acceptable control. Home monitoring of blood glucose (Dextrostix, Chemstrip bG, etc.) is especially helpful in planning therapy. Finger puncture with disposable lancets using an automatic, spring-loaded apparatus (Autolet, Autoclick, etc.) facilitates blood sampling and is practically painless. The reagent strips for checking the blood glucose are reliable when care is taken to follow directions but they cost $40-50/100 strips. If the patient can not afford this method of monitoring their diabetes, then urine is checked before meals and at bedtime on a "double-void" specimen (empty bladder first, then urinate 15-30 min later and check this specimen) using either tablets (Clinitest 2 drop method) or reagent strips. The goal for control is aglycosuria with very infrequent insulin reactions.

In most patients with "brittle" diabetes, one injection of an intermediate-acting insulin will not control the blood sugar throughout the day. Increasing the dose to > 60 U day as a single injection greatly increases the risk of hypoglycemia. To avoid these problems we split the insulin into two injections of intermediate insulin (before breakfast; before the evening meal) and add a short-acting insulin (regular, Semilente, or Actrapid). In theory, it is possible to "cover" the entire 24 hr day with such a "split-mixed" regimen. A patient whose blood glucose changes over time is used to demonstrate how insulin might be used:

Initially the blood sugars were acceptable on a single dose of 25 U NPH insulin each morning. Now while taking 30 U of NPH U-100 each AM, his blood sugars (mg/dl) for 3 consecutive days are as follows:

Breakfast	Lunch	Dinner	Bedtime
140	250	110	115
100	300	130	120
95	300	125	80

There is consistent hyperglycemia prior to lunch. If regular insulin were added to the NPH injection before breakfast, then the short-acting effect (3-4 hr peak) should cover the period of hyperglycemia derived from the meal at breakfast. Therefore, we add 5-10 U of regular insulin to the 30 U NPH q AM. Both insulins can be drawn up in one syringe and given as a single injection (first drawing up regular and then the NPH to avoid contamination of regular with NPH). The patient should be instructed to rotate (use different areas) his sites of insulin injection and to continue monitoring his blood sugar to see if the change helped lower the blood sugar prior to lunch.

After six months, this patient while taking 30 U NPH and 5 U regular q AM presents with blood sugars (mg/dl) on three consecutive days as follows:

Breakfast	Lunch	Dinner	Bedtime
300	140	90	110
270	135	120	85
310	125	130	100

Since the blood sugars are all > 150 mg/dl prior to breakfast, there are two possibilities to be considered. First, we ask if there is evidence for nocturnal hypoglycemia (awake with headache, wet bedclothes, "bad" dreams, or obvious insulin reaction)? If there is evidence for hypoglycemia, then the morning hyperglycemia (or glucosuria) probably reflects the counter-regulatory response to prior hypoglycemia (Somogyi phenomenon). In such a case we would decrease the morning NPH by 10-15% to 25 U. If there is no evidence for hypoglycemia, then we assume that the AM NPH is not covering the last 8 hrs of the 24 hr clock. The best way to correct this is to give NPH 30-60 min prior to the evening meal. Start with 5 U and add more if the hyperglycemia persists. Nocturnal reactions are likely to occur when large single doses of NPH are given or when the NPH before the evening meal is excessive. As before, the patient is responsible for monitoring and recording his glucose values.

In cases where there is persistent hyperglycemia prior to bedtime, then we can add regular insulin (2-10 U) prior to the evening meal which should cover that meal and reduce the bedtime hyperglycemia. The combination of NPH and regular insulin taken twice daily is called a "split-mixed" program and offers the advantage of providing insulin thoughout the 24-hr day as well as the convenience of taking only 2 injections/day and considerable flexibility in controlling hyperglycemia without producing hypoglycemia (fig. 3.1).

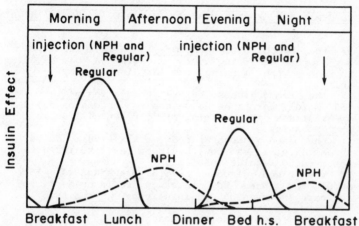

Figure 3.1 Split-Mixed Program of Twice a Day Insulin. Regular and intermediate insulin are taken together as a single injection 30-60 min prior to breakfast and to the evening meal.

Patients on a single dose of NPH insulin (45-60+ U/day) who are having hyperglycemia as well as hypoglycemic reactions are empirically changed to a split-mixed program. A total daily dose is selected (0.7 U/kg); let's say 60 U in an example case. Generally 2/3 of the total dose (40 U) is given in the morning (before breakfast) and the remaining 1/3 prior to the evening meal (20 U). The ratios are 2/3 intermediate-acting insulin and 1/3 regular in the morning and 1/2 intermediate and 1/2 regular in the evening. Thus, in our example the morning insulin dose consists 27 U NPH and 13 U regular while the evening dose is 10 U NPH and 10 U regular. Care is taken to insure the patient's meals are regular, activity is coordinated with proper diet, and the patient understands the basic principles of treating his or her diabetes.

Education is the most important facet of long-term diabetic management. Written instructions to the patient and family are essential. Handouts containing recommendations for diabetic management (see Appendix, page 155) and algorithms such as the ones given below [courtesy of G.J. Ellis, M.D.] are very helpful in allowing patients to adjust their own split-mixed program and thereby to become responsible for their own diabetes care on a day-to-day basis.

HYPERGLYCEMIA NOT EXPLAINED BY UNUSUAL DIET/EXERCISE/INSULIN

If the blood glucose before lunch is > 150 mg/dl for three days in a row, begin on day 4 to increase the morning regular insulin by _____ units.

If the blood glucose before the evening meal is > 150 mg/dl for three days in a row, begin on day 4 to increase the morning NPH (or Lente) insulin by _____ units.

If the blood glucose at bedtime is > 150 mg/dl for three days in a row, begin on day 4 to increase the evening regular insulin by _____ units.

If the blood glucose before breakfast is > 150 mg/dl for three days in a row, begin on day 4 to increase the evening NPH insulin by _____ units.

Small changes of 1-5 units of each insulin (usually 10% of each dose) are written in the blanks and a copy of the algorithm given to the patient. For the patient who does not monitor his or her blood sugar, then urine sugars are monitored and the statement would read "If urine sugars are positive (record in %) before ..., then increase appropiate insulin by 5-10% for each % spill..."

HYPOGLYCEMIA NOT EXPLAINED BY UNUSUAL DIET/EXERCISE/INSULIN

For hypoglycemic reactions occurring between breakfast and lunch, reduce next morning's regular insulin by _____ units.

For hypoglycemic reactions occurring between lunch and the evening meal, reduce next morning's NPH (or Lente) by _____ units.

For hypoglycemic reactions occurring between evening meal and bedtime, reduce the next evening's regular insulin by _____ units.

For hypoglycemic reactions occuring between bedtime and breakfast, reduce the evening's NPH (or Lente) by _____ units.

Again small changes of 1-5 U (10% of dose) are filled in the blanks for the patient. Each patient should treat an insulin reaction at the onset of symptoms with fruit juice (4-8 oz.).

If the individual is a jogger or bicyclist, then insulin should be injected into the deltoid or abdominal areas rather than the thigh to avoid rapid absorption of the insulin and possible hypoglycemia.

Insulin pumps are becoming a practical (though expensive) mode of giving insulin over the entire 24-hr period as well as of giving boluses of insulin prior to meals. Although highly promoted by the manufacturers, the indications for and an advantages of pump therapy vs conventional split-mixed combination are unclear.

Complications of Insulin Therapy: Complications that relate directly to insulin administration include hypoglycemia, insulin-induced lipodystrophy, insulin resistance, and insulin allergy.

Hypoglycemia is the most frequent complication of insulin treatment. Recurrent hypoglycemia may be due to 1) omission or delay of meals; 2) unusual heavy exercise; 3) chronic insulin overdosage; or 4) errors in insulin administration or technique. These problems are identified by careful history taking and observation of injection technique, and are minimized by patient education. The Somogyi phenomenon (hypoglycemia followed by rebound hyperglycemia) should be suspected in patients who have urine glucoses that vary from negative to strongly positive with ketones within the same 24 hr day, and in patients who gain weight despite heavy glycosuria. Monitoring the blood sugar frequently over a 24 hr period is the best way to confirm this problem. If a 10-15% reduction of insulin given as a single injection does not produce adequate control of the blood sugar, one should change to a split-dose regimen.

·The immediate treatment of hypoglycemia is with oral carbohydrate (4-8 oz of sweentened drink). If the patient is unconscious, administer intravenous glucose (50 ml of 50% dextrose) or glucagon (1 mg intramuscularly). Dextrose 50 % is painful when given iv and should be reserved for the unconscious patient. If glucagon is used and the patient does not respond within 15 min, administer dextrose 50% since it is unlikely that a second dose of glucagon will be effective.

Lipodystropy relates to atropy or hypertropy of fat at the site of insulin injection. Lipoatropy is the most frequent and occurs commonly in young females. The reaction is due to immune complex formation with less purified insulins and is seen less frequently since the introduction of purer insulin preparations. Lipoatrophy usually resolves within 6-9 months after changing to highly purified insulin which is injected into periphery of the atrophied area. Repeated injections into the same area causes lipohypertrophy ("insulin tumors"). Frequent rotation of injection sites avoids this problem.

Insulin resistance, defined as a daily insulin requirement of more than 200 U for several days in the absence of ketoacidosis, infection, pregnancy, or an associated endocrinopathy (e.g., acromegaly, Cushing's syndrome, hyperthyroidism), can be divided into three categories: 1) immunogenic insulin resistance (the most common); 2) insulin receptor abnormalities (rare); and 3) local degradation of insulin (rare).

Immunogenic insulin resistance is associated with high titers of anti-insulin IgG antibodies to beef insulin and less often to pork insulin. Substitution to a highly purified pork insulin often proves effective. If this does not work, a two to three week course of glucocorticoids (prednisone 60-80 mg/day) may be tried. Since this regimen may increase resistance to insulin, worsen the hyperglycemia, and has complications inherent to high-dose glucocorticoids, it is best to demonstrate high titers of anti-insulin antibodies prior to instituting steroids (i.e., prove immunologic insulin resistance), and then manage the patient initially as an inpatient.

Insulin receptor abnormalities are associated with acanthosis nigricans (velvety, hyperpigmented areas of skin usually seen around the neck, in the axilla, and in the groin). Anti-insulin antibodies are not present. Two clinical syndromes related to a receptor abnormality are recognized: Type A and Type B. Type A (reduced number of insulin receptors) affects younger females with signs of virilization and accelerated growth related to ovarian androgen overproduction. Type B (antibodies to insulin receptor) affects older women with other signs of immunologic disease such as arthritis, leucopenia, and anti-nuclear antibodies.

Insulin resistance due to the local degradation of subcutaneous administrated insulin and normal sensitivity to intravenous insulin is easily diagnosed by a trial of low-dose intravenous insulin.

Insulin allergy presents usually as a local skin reaction and rarely as a systemic reaction. Local reactions are manifest as induration, erythema, and pruritus at the injection site within 30 min to 4 hr of insulin administration and are most likely to occur in patients who have recently started insulin therapy. This relates to an IgG-mediated response and resolves spontaneously in most patients after several weeks of continuous insulin therapy. For localized reactions that persist or become more severe, one changes to a purified pork insulin. A localized reaction with formation of subcutaneous nodules may be due to preservative (phenol) or zinc within the insulin preparation. Systemic insulin reactions are manifest by generalized pruritus and urticaria, angioedema, or acute anaphylaxis. Systemic reactions can be anticipated by the worsening of local reactions and are most likely to occur in patients who have had prior exposure to insulin but discontinued it temporarily. Treatment with desensitization as an inpatient with appropiate preparation to handle life-threatening anaphylaxis is mandatory. Desensitization is facilitated by a kit available from Eli Lilly Co., Indianapolis, IN.

Insulin in Type II diabetes: Although some patients with Type II diabetes require insulin, the very nature of the defect (insulin resistance and altered insulin secretory dynamics) usually means that insulin supplementation is not the answer to their hyperglycemia. Insulin therapy in these patients is an admission of therapeutic failure since what most of these patients need is weight reduction. The emphasis in Type II diabetes mellitus should be on diet and weight loss as primary therapy. Prescribing insulin leads to a vicious circle in which insulin lowers blood glucose, stimulates appetite, and promotes weight gain leading to more insulin resistance and finally a return to hyperglycemia. One clear indication for insulin treatment in Type II diabetes is to cover the acute stress situations such as surgery, infection, myocardial infarction, etc.

Oral hypoglycemic agents: Sulfonylurea drugs may be used to treat the hyperglycemia in Type II diabetes, but again use of these agents in the non-compliant obese subject is usually doomed to fail. Up to 60% of the patients have an initial good response of blood glucose but sulfonylureas produce effective long-term results in only 20-30% of patients. The failure rate plus the controversial UGDP findings (tolbutamide and phenformin increase cardiovascular mortality) have tempered the enthusiasm for the use of the current sulfonylureas. Each of the sulfonylureas available in the United States (tolbutamide, acetohexamide, tolazamide, and chlorpropamide) appears equally effective. The usual daily dose of tolbutamide is 500-1000 mg bid; acetohexamide, 250-500 mg bid; tolazamide, 250-1000 q d; and chlorpropamide, 100-500 mg q d. One must be alert however that chlorpropamide's prolonged duration of action (24-60 hrs) increases the risk of hypoglycemia. Chlorpropamide also may augment the release of vasopressin (ADH) leading to hyponatremia and possible water intoxication.

Exercise: Exercise is important in weight control and in modulating insulin dosage in diabetes mellitus. Exercise itself has a glucose-lowering effect. However, in the ketotic and severely hyperglycemic patient, exercise will worsen the hyperglycemia. Obese patients especially are encouraged to walk 3-5 miles per day to aid in weight reduction.

Glycosylated hemoglobin: Nonenzymatic addition of glucose to proteins forming stable glycoproteins is favored whenever the glucose concentration is high. Hemoglobin A is glycosylated to form hemoglobin A1 which normally represents less than 6% of the hemoglobin. In poorly controlled diabetics hemoglobin A1 accounts for > 12% of the total hemoglobin. The advantage of glycosylated hemoglobin measurement is that it correlates with glycemia during the last 6-8 weeks (half-life of erythrocyte is about 120 days) and gives an integrated value in contrast to blood sugar which fluctuates widely. The disadvantage of glycosylated hemoglobin is that the assay is difficult and standards are not available to compare various assay techniques. When properly performed the glycosylated hemoglobin is helpful in confirming whether the control of blood sugar has been "on the average" what the patient says it has been. Whether glycosylation of proteins in general has any direct role in the pathogenesis of diabetic complications (micro- or macro-vascular disease) is uncertain.

Surgery and The Diabetic:

There are a number of methods to cover the diabetic who needs general surgery. It is important, regardless of the regimen used, that the patient's blood sugars monitored frequently. Fingerstick blood glucose, recorded at the bedside, is rapid and convenient. The frequency of blood glucose checks must to be individualized. Good preoperative control of the diabetes will make elective surgery and anesthesia management much easier. Uncontrolled diabetes coupled with the stress of surgery may progress to ketoacidosis or hyperosmolar coma.

Most patients are kept fasting after midnight prior to surgery. Intravenous 5% dextrose solution, 100-150 ml/hr, is started around dawn and regular insulin given subcutaneously. The amount and route of insulin administration depend on the patient's normal <u>total</u> daily insulin dose and the type of surgery. The total daily dose is divided by 4. This value is given as regular insulin sc q 6 hrs as long as iv's are infusing. The first dose is given usually at 7-8 AM on the day of surgery. This regimen is used for all surgery except those operations requiring hypothermia (e.g., cardiac) where absorption may be erratic. In these special situations regular insulin is given as a continuous iv drip at 1 U/hr. The rate is increased or decreased according to fingersticks blood glucose. Blood sugars between 100-200 mg/dl are acceptable.

Postoperative orders using urine glucose for "a sliding scale insulin" dose are a surgical tradition but one that should be avoided. Since the renal threshold for glucose must be exceeded before any glycosuria is detected, the "sliding scale" treats hyperglycemia "after the fact," and doesn't offer a means of preventing hyperglycemia. Poor wound healing is associated with the greater degree of glycemia. A better regimen maintains the q 6 hr insulin program and supplements the doses with additional regular insulin in amounts based on the blood glucose. Additional regular insulin is added to the q 6 hr insulin using an algorithm based on the blood sugar just prior to scheluded injection (the advantage of fingersticks and reflectometer readings at bedside is obvious). For blood sugars between 200 and 250 mg/dl, add 2-4 U; between 251 and 300, add 3-6 U; and for blood sugars > 300, add 5-10 U. The exact extra amount is varied depending on the basal dose with the larger amounts being used for patients receiving larger basal doses. If the basal amount needs constant supplementation, then the basal dose is raised; if the blood sugar is low (< 60 mg/dl), then the basal dose is reduced.

As soon as the patient can eat, regular insulin is given before meals and before bedtime with a bedtime snack. No more than 10 U are given hs to avoid nocturnal hypoglycemia. Alternatively the prior normal insulin program may be reinstituted and regular insulin added for ac blood sugars > 200 mg/dl. The importance of monitoring the sugar and making day to day adjustments can not be overemphasized.

References

Clements RS Jr: Diabetic neuropathy--new concepts of its etiology. Diabetes 28:604, 1979.

Felig P: The endocrine pancreas: diabetes mellitus, in Felig P, Baxter JD, Broadus AE, Frohman LA (eds): Endocrinology and Metabolism. New York, McGraw-Hill, 1981, pp 761-868.

Flier JS, Kahn CR, Roth J: Receptors, antireceptor antibodies, and mechanisms of insulin resistance. N Engl J Med 300:413, 1979.

Gabbay KH: Childhood diabetes mellitus, in Krieger DT, Bardin CW (eds): Current Therapy in Endocrinology 1983-1984. Burlington, Ontario, BC Decker, 1983, pp 154-160.

Galloway JA, Bressler R: Insulin treatment in diabetes. Med Clin North Am 62:663, 1978.

Jarrett J: Diabetes and the heart: coronary artery disease. Clin Endocrinol Metabol 6:389, 1977.

Kohner EM: Diabetic retinopathy. Clin Endocrinol Metab 6:345, 1977.

Koenig RJ, Peterson CM, Jones RL, Saudek C, Lehrman M, Cerami A: Correlation of glucose regulation and hemoglobin A1c in diabetes mellitus. N Engl J Med 295:417, 1976.

Lebovitz HE, Feinglos MN: Sulfonylurea drugs: mechanism of antidiabetic action and therapeutic usefulness. Diabetes Care 1:189, 1978.

National Diabetes Data Group: Classification and diagnosis of diabetes mellitus and other categories of glucose intolerance. Diabetes 28:1039, 1979.

Shuman CR: The adult diabetic patient, in Krieger DT, Bardin CW (eds): Current Therapy in Endocrinology 1983-1984. Burlington, Ontario, BC Decker, 1983, pp 160-169.

Sonksen PH, Judd SL, Lowy C: Home monitoring of blood glucose. Method for improving diabetic control. Lancet 1:729, 1979.

Chapter 4

Hypoglycemia

Hypoglycemia is defined operationally as a blood glucose low enough to produce neuroglycopenic and/or homeostatic (adrenergic) symptoms. Neuroglycopenia is manifest by inability to concentrate, confusion, incoherent speech, headache, blurred vision, bizarre behavior, focal or generalized seizures, stupor, coma, and finally death. Homeostatic symptoms relate to the sympathomimetic stimulation of hormones including epinephrine, norepinephrine, cortisol, glucagon, and growth hormone which will raise blood glucose in response to hypoglycemia. These homeostatic responses produce the most striking symptoms including sweating, palpitations, hunger, tremor, tachycardia, and anxiety. These are the early warning signs of hypoglycemia whereas most of the neuroglycopenic symptoms occur when the hypoglycemia is more profound. Two other characteristics of hypoglycemic symptoms are their episodic nature and relief of symptoms with glucose ingestion. Each episode of hypoglycemic symptoms will last for minutes to hours because either counter-regulatory responses will spontaneously raised plasma glucose or the patient will eat food to raise the plasma glucose. However relief of symptoms with food or beverage does not make a diagnosis of hypoglycemia since this is not specific for hypoglycemia.

Several factors determine whether a particular level of glucose will produce symptoms. Sex is a factor since healthy females have a 10-15 mg/dl lower plasma glucose level than males during a 72 hr fast. The antecedent level of plasma glucose is also important since diabetic patients with chronic hyperglycemia may manifest hypoglycemic symptoms at plasma glucose 90-100 mg/dl whereas normal subjects with glucoses raise acutely to 300 mg/dl then reduced abruptly will not have any symptoms until the plasma glucose is reduced to < 50 mg/dl. The rapidity of plasma glucose fall may determine whether symptoms will occur, but the level of blood/plasma glucose itself is the most critical parameter in whether symptoms will develop. Confusion may exist if one is not aware of whether the values are reported in terms of blood glucose or plasma glucose. Most glucose determinations are now measured on plasma which will have about 15% more glucose/volume than blood glucose determinations (RBC's occupy space so there is less glucose/volume in blood).

A diagnosis of hypoglycemia is made when the patient has the symptoms listed above _and_ plasma glucose levels < 60 mg/dl after overnight fast in both males and females or < 50 mg/dl on an oral glucose tolerance test or < 45 mg/dl for females and < 55 mg/dl for males after a 72 hr fast. Symptoms alone do not make a diagnosis of hypoglycemia since most of these reflect nonspecific increase in adrenergic discharge nor do low plasma glucoses alone establish the diagnosis of hypoglycemia _unless_ there are accompanying neuroglycopenic or homeostatic symptoms. Much confusion regarding hypoglycemia can be avoided if these criteria for the diagnosis are met.

Clinically hypoglycemia can be grouped into three major categories: induced, fasting, and postprandial hypoglycemia. Induced or exogenous hypoglycemia is by far the most common and is caused by the administration of medication (insulin, sulfonylureas, salicylates) or ingestion of toxic chemicals (alcohol). Fasting hypoglycemias may be caused by endocrine disease (insulinomas, extra-pancreatic tumors, adrenal insufficiency, pituitary insufficiency), hepatic disorders (glycogen storage disease, deficiency of gluconeogenic enzymes, acute hepatic necrosis), or rarely substrate deficiency in which the liver cannot produce enough glucose from lack of precursors (fasting hypoglycemia of pregnancy, ketotic hypoglycemia of childhood, uremia, and starvation). Postprandial or reactive hypoglycemia is the catch-all category characterized by hypoglycemic symptoms (adrenergic type) that develop with a few hours of eating (idiopathic reactive hypoglycemia, hereditary fructose intolerance).

Induced hypoglycemias do not require an exhausting workup, but a carefully taken history is mandatory. For the diabetic with insulin reactions these are pertinent questions: Is the current dosage excessive? Did the patient miss a meal or regular snack? Were no changes made for rigorous work or exercise? Was the injection technique correct--intramuscular vs subcutaneous (im is likely to have rapid absorption and possible hypoglycemia), runner or bicyclist injecting thigh vs abdomen (insulin is absorbed rapidly from an exercising limb and should be taken in the abdominal wall in these instances)? Are reactions related to developing adrenal or pituitary insufficiency? Is the patient developing renal insufficiency? Is the diabetic taking propranolol or developing autonomic neuropathy that may mask the early adrenergic symptoms of hypoglycemia? For the diabetic taking sulfonylurea agents similar questions

are appropiate: Has the patient just started on oral agents
(the time when hypoglycemia with these agents is most likely
to develop)? Is the patient developing renal insufficiency
while taking chlorpropamide or acetohexamide (drugs that are
secreted by kidneys)? Is the patient taking other
medication which might potentiate the hypoglycemic actions
of sulfonylureas (salicylates, phenylbutazone,
sulfisoxazole)? Alcohol-induced hypoglycemia develops in
subjects whose livers have been depleted of glycogen and
therefore is seen in malnourished individuals or in subjects
who have fasted for 48-72 hrs while imbibing alcohol. This
is typically seen in binge drinkers. Hypoglycemia develops
6-24 hrs after drinking ceases. These patients often
present with hypothermia, coma, plasma glucoses (< 30
mg/dl), tachypnea (lactic acidosis), with or without ethanol
on breath, blood ethanol levels below acute intoxication,
and abnormal liver function studies. These patients do not
have a hyperglycemic response when given intramuscular
injection of glucagon.

Fasting hypoglycemia is more difficult to diagnose by
history than induced hypoglycemia. Because this condition
is associated with significant pathology, the workup should
be complete and the diagnosis definitive. By definition
these patients fail to maintain plasma glucose homeostasis
when food is withheld. The most common fasting hypoglycemia
is factitious. These patients will have low plasma glucoses
and high insulins as the patients with insulinoma. They
surreptitiously inject insulin or ingest oral hypoglycemic
agents and present for management as fasting hypoglycemia
even though they really fall into the induced hypoglycemia
category. Paramedical individuals (nurses, pharmacists,
etc) or relatives of diabetic patients are suspect for this
problem. A diligent search for needle marks and hospital
room for insulin/sulfonylureas is well worth the effort as
is telephoning previous physicians/hospitals. If the
patient has been injecting insulin for several months, the
serum insulin levels may appear be very high (> 500 uU/ml)
secondary to antibody formation which interferes with the
insulin RIA measurement. Assaying for C-peptide (the
connecting peptide of proinsulin which is released in the
same molar equivalents as insulin) is helpful in factitious
insulin abuse where the level will be low, but C-peptide
levels are not helpful in sulfonylurea abuse where the
levels will be high. Urinary screening for sulfonylureas
should be positive in these instances.

Patients with insulin-producing pancreatic islet adenomas
(insulinomas) and tumors arising outside the pancreas
classically present with fasting hypoglycemia. Insulinomas
are typically seen in the middle aged (> 30 yrs)

individual. The most important question to answer is the time of hypoglycemic symptoms. Headache prior to breakfast or the appearance of symptoms after exercise suggest fasting hypoglycemia. Weight gain oftens occurs since food is eaten frequently to abort or relieve the symptoms. A family history of multiple endocrine adenomatosis should be sought.

The diagnosis of insulinoma is made when the fasting plasma glucose is low and the plasma insulin inappropiately elevated. Insulin (uU/ml) over glucose (mg/dl) ratio is normally < 0.25; a ratio > 0.3 is generally indicative of hyperinsulinism. Most patients with an insulinoma will manifest hypoglycemia within 18 hrs after eating. In those patients who don't manifest symptoms early and in those whose symptoms cannot be discerned from reactive hypoglycemia, an inpatient fast of 72 hrs is indicated. Ad lib water is given and urine ketones monitored. Monitoring urine ketones is a good bedside study since it is very unlikely the patient will have hyperinsulinism if the ketones are positive because insulin inhibits lipolysis. Plasma glucose and insulin are drawn every 6 hr or more often if symptoms arise. C-peptide levels should be elevated with an insulinoma. Plasma glucoses < 45 mg/dl and insulins > 6 uU/ml are diagnostic of hyperinsulinism.

The treatment is surgical removal of the tumor. Selective mesenteric arteriography can help locate the tumor, but the surgeon's skill and expertise are really the most critical factor. In one series from the Mayo Clinic (154 patients) there was a 5.4% operative mortality and in over 10% of the cases the tumor was not found at surgery. Diazoxide may be tried in patients who refuse surgery or those whose hyperinsulinism was not cured by surgery. Metastatic islet cell tumors do respond to streptozotocin but the response is unfortunately not curative by any means.

Large mesothelial derived tumors (retroperitoneal fibrosarcomas, hemangiopericytomas), hepatomas, and adrenal carcinomas may present with fasting hypoglycemia. These tumors are large and generally easily palpable as abdominal masses. The mechanism by which the tumors cause hypoglycemia is unknown. Insulin levels are low. In some patients (40 %) radioimmunoassayable insulin-like growth factor (IGF) is elevated. The tumor may overutilize glucose because of sheer bulk, but most likely some product is released which inhibits hepatic gluconeogenesis/ glycogenolysis.

Antibodies to the insulin receptor typically block insulin action leading to hyperglycemia (see immunogenic insulin resistance, page 48). However, antibodies to the insulin receptor may rarely stimulate glucose transport leading to hypoglycemia. Other evidence of autoimmune response is also present (e.g., anti-nuclear antibodies, rheumatoid factor, etc.).

Postprandial hypoglycemia can be diagnosed when the symptoms of hypoglycemia are associated temporally with plasma glucoses < 50 mg/dl after a meal. In a subset of patients who have had gastric surgery, alimentary hypoglycemia appears to be due to excessive glucose loads within the duodenum which leads to quick absorption and rapid release of insulin with resultant fall of plasma glucose to a nadir within 2.5 hrs after feeding. Small frequent feedings, avoidance of foods with high simple sugar content, and judicious use of anticholinergic medication is helpful.

Idiopathic or reactive hypoglycemia is diagnosed using the same criteria as for postprandial hypoglycemia. The nadir occurs between 3 and 4 hrs after feeding with a return to normal fasting values by the 5th and 6th hr. If there is no rebound to normal values, then a workup to exclude fasting hypoglycemia (insulinoma, adrenal or pituitary insufficiency) should be considered. The number of individuals who have this benign syndrome of idiopathic reactive hypoglycemia is exceeding small. These patients respond to a low carbohydrate (120 gm), relatively high protein diet given as 6 feedings throughout the day.

Many patients make their own diagnosis of reactive hypoglycemia, attributing the symptoms of adrenergic discharge, mental and physical fatigue, and weakness that may or may not be relieved by glucose-laden food or beverage to "hypoglycemia." The lay press and media have fanned the fires by popularizing this "entity". Physicians have confused the issue themselves by not having a study that can mimic the conditions which these patients have symptoms. The time-honored oral glucose tolerance test (GTT) has many problems. At least 24% of healthy inductees into the service have 2 hr plasma glucose < 60 mg/dl, and 5% have plasma glucose < 50 mg/dl without any symptoms. In another study of 650 patients who had no symptoms before or during GTT, 10% had plasma glucose values < 47 mg/dl. The frequency of biochemical hypoglycemia is the same for patients who present for evaluation of reactive hypoglycemia as it is for the normal population. In addition most of the patients being evaluated for hypoglycemia with the GTT have symptoms when the corresponding plasma glucoses are in the normal range. The 75-100 gm load of glucose is not a physiological challenge since this is not what subjects eat at meals. These factors make interpreting the GTT results difficult. The GTT has a place in making a diagnosis of diabetes mellitus but its use in evaluating hypoglycemia is very questionable. An attempt to use mixed meals (1/4-1/3 total daily calories distributed as 50% CHO::20% protein::30% fat) as a challenge that might precipitate symptoms that these patients complain has shown that those patients who have biochemical hypoglycemia on a GTT do not have low plasma glucose after a mixed meal yet have the same adrenergic symptoms. Thus, low plasma glucoses can not be confirmed to be related to 95+% of patient in whom the diagnosis of reactive hypoglycemia is tentatively made.

The hordes of patients with "non-hypoglycemic hypoglycemia" or "pseudohypoglycemia" that present to the endocrinologist's practice with the diagnosis of reactive hypoglycemia is astounding. What to say and what to recommend to these people who are looking for a handle to label their symptoms and a means of controlling these symptoms requires clinical discernment. All of these patients (most often females ages 20-45) have stresses either recognized or not acknowledged. Many have chronic fatigue and somatic complaints lasting days and weeks that do not conform to typical episodic spells of true hypoglycemia. How well these patients are handling stress is reflected in the "hypoglycemic" symptoms. A tender ear and a soft tongue giving an honest assessment of the particular situation is a beginning step in managing these patients. A 120 gm carbohydrate diet low in simple sugars and instructions from an innovative dietician are helpful and should be prescibed. For the recalcitrant patient who has failed to improve despite discussion and diet, psychiatric referral may be helpful.

References

Charles MA, Hofeldt F, Shackelford A, Waldeck N, Dodson LE Jr, Bunker D, Coggins JT, Eichner H: Comparison of oral glucose tolerance tests and mixed meals in patients with apparent idiopathic postabsorptive hypoglycemia: absence of hypoglycemia after meals. Diabetes 30:465, 1981.

Ensinck JW: Postprandial hypoglycemia, in Kreiger DT, Bardin CW (eds): Current Therapy in Endocrinology 1983-1984. Burlington, Ontario, BC Decker, 1983, pp 215-222.

Hogan MJ, Service FJ, Sharbrough FW, Gerich JE: Oral glucose tolerance test compared with a mixed meal in the diagnosis of reactive hypoglycemia: a caveat on stimulation. Mayo Clin Proc 58:491, 1983.

Johnson DD, Dorr KE, Swenson WM, Service J: Reactive hypoglycemia. JAMA 243:1151,1980.

Laroche GP, Ferris DO, Priestley JT, Scholz DA, Dockerly MR: Hyperinsulinism: surgical results and management of occult functioning islet cell tumors; review of 154 cases. Arch Surg 96:763, 1968.

Lev-Ran A, Anderson RW: The diagnosis of postprandial hypoglycemia. Diabetes 30:996, 1981.

Sherwin RS, Felig P: Hypoglycemia, in Felig P, Baxter JD, Broadus AE, Frohman LA (eds): Endocrinology and Metabolism. New York, McGraw-Hill, 1981, pp 869-889.

Taylor SI, Grunberger G, Marcus-Samuels B, Underhill LH et al: Hypoglycemia associated with antibodies to the insulin receptor. N Engl J Med 307:1422, 1982.

Chapter 5

Pituitary Disease

Patients with pituitary-hypothalamic disorders present because of symptoms of a mass lesion (i.e., headaches, blindness, visual field defect), because of hypersecretion of a tropic hormone (prolactinoma, acromegaly, Cushing's disease), because of loss of tropic hormone(s) (hypopituitarism) or because of some combination of these.

Mass lesion: A mass lesion of the pituitary or hypothalmus should be suspected in several circumstances: 1) Enlarged sella turcica on skull X-ray, 2) Neurological symptoms and signs (headaches and/or loss of vision), or 3) endocrine disorders of the pituitary or hypothalamus. The most common question regarding a mass lesion is whether enlargement of the sella turcica is related to any endocrine disorder. A chance or serenpiditous finding of an enlarged sella turcica on skull roentgenographs obtained for a variety of reasons (trauma, sinusitis, headache, etc.) is not uncommon. The sella is considered enlarged if the length from the most anterior convexity to the most posterior aspect of the sella is > 17 mm and if the height from the floor to a line drawn between the anterior and posterior clinoid processes is > 13 mm. Other equally important roentgenographic signs are: configuration of the sella; evidence of bony erosion; and presence of suprasellar calcification. If there is no obvious endocrine or visual disorder, it is most likely that the enlarged sella turcica is an empty sella. During pneumoencephalography the sella fills with air and only a remnant of pituitary gland can be demonstrated. Pituitary function studies in these patients are generally normal. Patients with primary empty sella (i.e., not a result of surgery or radiation therapy) often share some common features: 84% are females, 78% are obese, 30% have elevated blood pressure, 10% have benign intracranial hypertension, and 10% have CSF rhinorrhea. There is herniation of CSF into the sella leading to uniform remodeling of the bone and the characteristic "ballooned" configuration seen in 84% of the patients. The diagnosis of empty sella is confirmed when the CT scan (or pneumoencephalogram) identifies no mass within an enlarged sella turcica. The CT scan demonstration of empty sella does not exclude small coexistent tumors hypersecreting growth hormone, or

prolactin, or ACTH. <u>No specific therapy is needed for the</u>
<u>empty sella.</u> The patient who presents with CSF rhinorrhea
or chiasmal syndrome due to herniation into an empty fossa
or with a hyperfunctioning microadenoma is treated by
conventional neurosurgical techniques.

Some mass lesions of the pituitary or hypothalamus present
solely with <u>neurologic symptoms.</u> The precise symptoms
depend on the location of the mass. Pituitary lesions are
likely to cause headache as the lesion expands against the
dura of the diaphragm of the sella. With progressive
superior extension of tumor the inferior optic chiasma is
compressed leading to a visual field cut in the macula
(detected by testing for color vision with a red dot-page
69), then to superior temporal field cut, then to classic
bitemporal hemianopsia and eventually to blindness. Visual
symptoms are less often a presenting complaint nowadays than
they were in the past, but this is still a common mode of
pituitary tumor presentation in older patients.

Papilledema is rare in pituitary tumors (which usually
cause optic atrophy) but is common in suprasellar tumors
such as craniopharyngiomas where up to one fourth of
patients have papilledema. Craniopharyngiomas are midline,
predominantly cystic tumors that develop at the upper end of
the pituitary stalk. These are tumors of youth since about
half of these patients are under 20 yrs of age.
Calcification in the suprasellar region occurs in > 50% of
patients. Craniopharyngiomas are much more likely to
compress midline hypothalamic structures leading to
neurological symptoms earlier than do pituitary tumors.
Diabetes insipidus is common with craniopharyngioma and rare
with pituitary tumors.

<u>Endocrinologic symptoms</u> are now the most common present-
ing complaints of patients with pituitary tumors. Hormonal
manifestations of pituitary tumors are caused by
hypersecretion of a pituitary hormone, or deficiency of
pituitary hormone(s) or a combination of excess and lack of
tropic hormones.

<u>Hypersecretion of a pituitary hormone:</u> The pituitary
secretes growth hormone (GH), gonadotropins (FSH and LH),
thyroid stimulating hormone (TSH), adrenocorticotropic
hormone (ACTH), vasopressin (ADH), and prolactin (hPr).
Tumors which hypersecrete each of these hormones have been
described but only those associated with hPR, GH, ACTH are
usually seen, the others being extremely rare.

Prolactin: Prolactin-secreting adenoma (prolactinoma) is the   most   common   pituitary   tumor   and   causes   menstrual irregularity,   amenorrhea,   infertility,   and   often galactorrhea   in   the   female   and   decreased   libido   and impotence   in   the   male.   Excess   prolactin   inhibits gonadotropin   secretion   leading to hypogonadism.   Generally there   is   a good correlation between tumor bulk size and the level   of   serum prolactin.   The diagnosis of prolactinoma is generally   assured   when the serum prolactin levels are > 200 ng/ml.   For   lesser   degrees   of elevation one should review the   possibility   of   other   causes   of   hyperprolactinemia including   drugs   (estrogens,   birth   control   pills, phenothiazines,   tricyclic   antidepressants,   opiates   and opioids,   cimetidine,   butyrophenones,   reserpine,   Aldomet, isoniazid);   hypothyroidism;   stress;   etc. (see page 14).   The CT   scan   is the best radiographic tool for demonstrating the tumor   but   very   small   lesions may not be visualized.   Most prolactinomas   do   not stain with routine histological stains and therefore have been called chromophobe adenomas.

Treatment   of   prolactinoma   is   constantly   evolving   and remains   controversial.   If   there   is   evidence   of   visual compromise,   most authorities recommend neurosurgical removal even   though   the chance of total extirpation of the tumor is low   (<   30% chance of restoring normal prolactin levels). If   the   patient   desires fertility and has a serum prolactin level   <   200   ng/dl and a localized lesion on CT, there is a 90%   chance   that   an   experienced   neurosurgeon   using   the transsphenoidal   approach   can   resect   the   microadenoma, preserve   normal   pituitary   function,   and   reduce the serum prolactin   to   normal.   For   women   who desire fertility and have   no   clear adenoma on CT and whose serum prolactin < 200 ng/dl,   treatment   with   the dopamine agonist, bromocriptine, is   likely   to normalized prolactin levels and produce ovulation.   Bromocriptine, 1.25 mg to 2.5 mg tid (start 1.25 mg   hs   to   reduce nausea),   is given until the pregnancy is confirmed,   and   then   bromocriptine   is discontinued.   Close attention   should   be   paid   to   visual   fields   since   the pituitary   lesion may occasionally enlarge during pregnancy. Bromocriptine   occasionally   decreases   the   size   of   a prolactinoma;   but,   in   general, its tumoricidal activity is low   since once bromocriptine is stopped, the serum prolactin returns   to   existing   levels   prior to therapy.   The expense for   long-term   administration   is   relatively   high ($.55-.80/2.5   mg   tab).   The FDA has approved bromocriptine for   infertility   and   chronic   idiopathic hyperprolactinemia (no   tumor)   for   a   six   month   course of therapy.   Another dopamine   agonist,   pergolide,   appears to be as effective as bromocriptine and has the advantage of once a day dose.

Males   with   hyperprolactinemia   usually   have   severe elevations   of   prolactin   and   often present with impotence and symptoms of a pituitary mass.   Resection of tumor and treatment of hypogonadism (page 83) is indicated.

Growth Hormone: Hypersecretion of growth hormone leads to _gigantism_ in children and to _acromegaly_ in adults. Growth hormone-secreting tumors stain eosinophilic in 20% of the cases and chromophobic in the remainder of the cases. The changes with acromegaly are subtle, slow, and progressive for years and lead to a dramatic clinical syndrome which is not easily confused with any other syndrome.   The effects of chronic hypersecretion of growth hormone are mediated through somatomedin.   This insulin-like growth factor causes tissue growth which is accentuated in the acral areas of the skeleton. The acral changes are most prominent in the hands where the fingers are broad and sausage-like.   A   handshake unmistakenly suggests acro- megaly in these patients.   The ring size, glove size, and shoe size have enlarged over the years.   The facial features are coarse with thick skin folds, furrowed brows, and prominent nasolabial creases.   The cartilage of the nose hypertrophies leading to nasal enlargement.   The mandible grows which gives an overbite, prognathism, and wide spaces between the teeth.   Skin changes include fibroma molluscum, sebaceous hypersecretion, and sebaceous cyst formation. These patients have increased sweating which improves as the activity of the disease subsides.   Bone overgrowth causes hypertrophic osteoarthropathy which is symptomatically one of the difficult problems to treat.   Carpal tunnel and other entrapment syndromes result from ligamentous hypertrophy. The liver, kidney, spleen, and salivary glands hypertrophy. Hypertension is common and needs vigorous treatment.   Overt diabetes mellitus is found in at least one fourth of these patients.   The serum T4(RIA) and testosterone levels are often low because the concentration of binding proteins for each of these hormones is lowered in acromegaly.

The diagnosis of acromegaly is confirmed by finding elevated fasting blood levels of GH (usually > 10 ng/ml) which do _not_ suppress with glucose (see pages 7 and 36) or are raised paradoxically in response to TRH (GH levels in normal subjects do not respond to TRH).   GH is elevated in chronic renal failure, starvation, and anorexia nervosa. Rare cases of ectopic production of GH or GH-releasing hormone have been reported in bronchial carcinoid and pancreatic islet cell tumor.

Acromegaly is treated with surgery or radiation and often with both.   Therapy has to be individualized for each patient and each medical center.   Those patients whose GH levels are > 100 ng/ml do not have great results with either surgery or radiation although GH levels may decrease dramatically and provide some clinical improvement.

Conventional supervoltage irradiation delivering 4500-5000 rads to the sella through multiple ports is safe but it takes months to years to lower GH levels. Radiation is recommended for acromegalic patients who have persistent non-suppressible GH levels after surgery. Response to treatment is assessed by measuring fasting or post-glucose GH levels. The bulk of clinical experience relates to GH rather than somatomedin measurements. GH levels are generally more available and are much less expensive than somatomedin C determinations.

ACTH: ACTH-producing pituitary tumors create a state of hypercortisolism which is clinically indistinguishable from other causes of glucocorticoid excess. By convention the association of bilateral adrenal hyperplasia with pituitary tumor is called Cushing's disease. Any clinical syndrome of glucocorticoid excess is called Cushing's syndrome. The most common cause of Cushing's syndrome is ingestion of pharmacological doses glucocorticoids for a variety of non-endocrine diseases.

ACTH-producing pituitary tumors are small and generally not detected by skull X-ray or CT scan. The symptoms of Cushing's syndrome lead to evaluation early in the course of the disease accounting for the infrequent radiographic findings. The tumor stains basophilic in 80% of the cases and chromophobic in the remainder (which lack the glycosylated form of ACTH form responsible for the basophilic staining). Plasma ACTH levels are modestly elevated but not enough to be of diagnostic help. The normal ACTH diurnal variation is lost but these results are difficult to decipher unless run under research conditions (see page 9).

The clinical signs of hypercortisolism include centripetal obesity with prominent supraclavicular fat pads, dorsal hump, and dewlap; muscle weakness and protein wasting with thin skin, facial plethora, bruising, and violaceous striae; hyperandrogenism with menstrual irregularity and hirsutism; back pain related to osteoporosis and compression fractures; hypertension particularly after the age of 40; and glucose intolerance or overt diabetes mellitus.

The first question to answer is whether an obese, hypertensive patient has hypercortisolism. An elevated urine cortisol will establish the diagnosis of Cushing's syndrome (see page 17). Once exogenous sources of glucocorticoids are excluded, the differential diagnosis of hypercortisolism is among Cushing's disease (70-80% of the cases), primary adrenal tumor either adenoma or carcinoma (10-15% of the cases), and ectopic production of ACTH by tumors (oat cell lung carcinomas, pancreatic islet cell carcinoma, thymoma, carcinoid tumors, medullary thyroid carcinoma, and neuroectodermal tumors). Dexamethasone suppression studies are used to separate the etiologies of the hypercortisolism (pages 11 and 12). Patients with Cushing's disease will suppress their adrenal steriod output as a result of ACTH suppression by high dose dexamethasone; patients with adrenal tumors and ectopic ACTH syndrome do not. The CT scan is very helpful in identifying adrenal masses. Oat cell carcinoma of the lung is the most frequent cause of ectopic ACTH syndrome. The clinical picture with ectopic ACTH is quite different than that of Cushing's disease or adrenal adenoma/carcinoma in that weight loss and electrolyte abnormalities with severe hypokalemia and alkalosis predominate. An occasional patient with ectopic ACTH may be confused with Cushing's disease if the clinical course is slow but dexamethasone suppression studies usually discriminate these cases.

In the past the only effective treatment of Cushing's disease was to remove the hypertrophied adrenal glands, leaving the patient permanently dependent on replacement glucocorticoid and mineralocorticoid. Significant hyperpigmentation and sella enlargement due to a large ACTH-producing tumor (Nelson's syndrome) followed adrenalectomy in about 8% of the cases. Transsphenoidal pituitary microsurgery, which can cure 85-95% of patients while preserving pituitary function, is the therapy of choice. However, these impressive results are not obtained in all centers and therefore the choice of therapy between transsphenoidal pituitary microsurgery or bilateral adrenalectomy will vary. Cyproheptadine, a serotonin antagonist, has occasionally produced amelioration of symptoms but generally the results with this therapy are poor. In children with Cushing's disease the treatment of choice is pituitary irradiation.

Deficiency of tropic hormones: Loss of tropic hormones leading to hypopituitarism is common in pituitary disorders. There are numerous and diverse causes including processes which may affect the pituitary directly leading to primary hypopituitarism (e.g., pituitary adenoma or hemorrhage) or indirectly by disturbing hypothalmus or stalk functions leading to secondary hypopituitarism (e.g., sarcoid). The following table lists most of the causes of hypopituitarism:

Table 5.1 Causes of Hypopituitarism

PRIMARY	SECONDARY
Pituitary tumors	Destruction of the stalk
Intrasellar and parasellar	Trauma
Infarction or ischemic necrosis	Compression by mass
Postpartum (Sheehan's syndrome)	Surgical transection
Shock	Hypothalmic disease
Sickle cell anemia	Inflammation (sarcoid)
Cavernous sinus thrombosis	Trauma
Carotid artery aneurysm or thrombosis	Toxic (vincristine)
Pituitary apoplexy	Hormone-Induced (high
Diabetes mellitus	glucocorticoids)
Inflammatory disease	Tumors
Meningitis (TB, fungal, malarial)	Functional
Pituitary abscess	Anorexia nervosa
Infiltrative disorders	Starvation
Hemochromatosis	Psychosocial dwarfism
Idiopathic	
Selective hormone deficiency	
Isolated GH deficiency	
Isolated ACTH deficiency	
Isolated TSH deficiency	
Hypogonadotropic hypogonadalism	
Multiple hormone deficiency	
Iatrogenic	
Irradiation to sella or nasopharynx	
Surgical destruction	

The clinical signs and symptoms of hypopituitarism relate to the underlying cause and to the specific tropic hormone(s) that are missing. The onset is usually insidious but occasionally the presentation is dramatic as with acute diabetes insipidus or pituitary apoplexy. Mass lesions compress and distort normal pituicytes leading to loss of tropic hormones. The tropic hormone usually lost first is growth hormone, followed by the gonadotropins, and finally by TSH and ACTH. ADH deficiency is rare with pituitary disease, but is common with stalk and hypothalmic lesions.

Growth hormone deficiency is not clinically detectable in the adult. In children GH deficiency leads to growth failure and short stature and rarely to hypoglycemia. Likewise gonadotropin deficiency causes no symptoms in the postmenopausal or post-hysterectomy female. Absence of FSH and LH produces hypogonadism with amenorrhea and infertility in adult females and impotence in adult males. Hypothyroidism secondary to TSH deficiency and hypoadrenalism secondary to ACTH deficiency are late complications of pituitary tumor. Patients with these deficiencies often present with a mass lesion and neurologic symptoms related to loss of vision. Isolated tropic hormone deficiency is usually diagnosed in youth because of failure to grow or failure to enter puberty.

Evaluation of pituitary hypofunction entails the following studies:

Static studies: Serum or urine taken for a single determination detect absolute deficiencies in some circumstances. For example, serum testosterone and LH are ordered in the evaluation of the impotent male. If both the testosterone and the LH are low, then these static studies establish the diagnosis of secondary hypogonadism. To completely evaluate the etiology of the hypogonadism several questions need to be addressed: 1) Are there other tropic hormone deficiencies? 2) Is the serum prolactin elevated (prolactin will suppress gonadotropin)? 3) Is there a mass lesion (visual fields compromised, abnormal sella turcica, enhanced lesion on CT scan)?

The following static studies are ordered to assess deficiencies of other pituitary hormones: ACTH is assessed indirectly by a 24 hr urine cortisol; TSH, by serum T4(RIA) and T3U; and ADH, by an early AM urine specific gravity. If any of the values are low in a patient with obvious pituitary disease, one can assume a deficiency for the appropiate tropic hormone.

STATIC STUDIES TO ASSESS PITUITARY HYPOFUNCTION		
Tropic Hormone	Study To Order	Hypopituitary Interpretation
GH	plasma growth hormone	low or normal (high in anorexia nervosa)
LH	if amenorrhea, serum LH if male, serum testosterone and serum LH	low LH (< 5 mIU/ml) low testosterone–low LH
FSH	serum FSH in women semen analysis and FSH for men	low FSH low sperm count and semen volume
TSH	T4(RIA) and T3U; serum TSH	low T4 and T3U; low TSH
ACTH	24 hr urine cortisol	low
hPr	serum prolactin	high (if prolactinoma)
ADH	early AM specific gravity	urine sp. gr. < 1.005

Serum prolactin should be determined since 70% of chromophobe adenomas secrete this hormone. Baseline prolactin values are helpful in planning follow-up therapy.

Visual fields should be assessed at the bedside and here the most reliable method is based on the patient's ability to count fingers shown by the examiner (fig. 5.1). The examiner asks the patient to look directly into the examiner's own pupil which allows comparison of the patient's visual field with that of the observer. With one eye occluded, either 1, 2, or 5 fingers are presented in each of four quadrants of the visual field in different positions and the patient is asked to give the correct number of fingers. Holding three and four fingers up are confusing and should be avoided. The majority of fibers in the optic chiasm derive from the central portion of the visual field and these axons subserve color vision. For this reason central visual fields are the first to be affected by expanding sellar tumors and can be tested using bright red objects (fig. 5.2). The patient fixates on the examiner's eye and is asked to compare the brightness of color of two objects, one held in the temporal field and the other held in the nasal field. Both objects are held together close to the line of fixation (central vision). In the case of a chiasmal lesion, the patient will be unable to distinguish the red color in the temporal field or will note that the test object is much redder in the nasal than in the temporal field.

Visual fields performed by perimetry (Goldmann apparatus) are important as a baseline study and is the procedure of choice for detecting minor visual field abnormalities and for following changes in visual fields. Testing of visual acuity is important and is a parameter that should not be neglected.

The CT scan is a powerful tool which has almost replaced the pneumoencephalogram in evaluation of mass lesions.

Dynamic studies: Serum or urine hormone concentration measured under stimulatory conditions can assess whether there is reserve for the respective hormone and ascertain whether the patient can tolerate surgical procedures or other stress situations. The insulin-induced hypoglycemia test is an ideal stimulatory study since both GH and cortisol can be measured (pages 7 and 8). Dynamic studies such as the insulin-induced hypoglycemia or metyrapone loading are not necessary in the patient with an obvious mass lesion. These studies are done primarily when there are questions as to whether there is any pituitary disease or dysfunction.

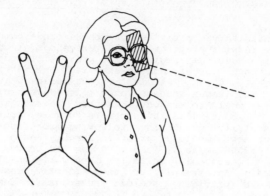

Figure 5.1   Visual fields by confrontation. With one eye
occluded, the patient fixates gaze on the examiner's eye.
The examiner asks the patient to enumerate 1, 2, or 5
fingers presented in each quadrant of the field. This exam
is repeated with the other eye occluded. [Neelon FA, Sydnor
CF: The assessment of pituitary function. Disease-a-Month
24(4):19, 1978. with permission]

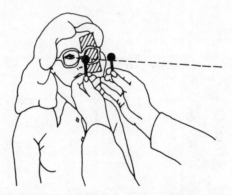

Figure   5.2   Assessing central visual fields by color
confrontation.   One eye is occluded and the patient gazes at
the examiner's pupil. Two bright objects (such as red paper
or bottle caps) are presented on both sides of fixation.
The patient is asked to compare presence and brightness of
color.   [Neelon FA, Syndor CF: The assessment of pituitary
function. Disease-a-Month 24(4):20, 1978. with permission]

MANAGING THE HYPOPITUITARY PATIENT DURING SURGICAL PROCEDURES

Hypopituitary patients or those undergoing pituitary surgery require preparation with exogenous glucocorticoids. There are several regimens to provide glucocorticoids for the stress of surgery and anesthesia. One method is to give Solu-Cortef 100 mg as intravenous drip q 6 hrs during surgery and taper the dose over a few days post-op until po meds are well tolerated. Another regimen which does not depend on continuous infusions is to give cortisone acetate intramuscularly using the following schelude: 100 mg into each buttock two days prior to surgery and on day prior to surgery (200 mg/day), and 100 mg im on call to the OR. Cortisone acetate 100 mg im is given daily until po meds are tolerated. An example of the effectiveness of such a regimen in providing steroid coverage is demonstrated in figure 5.3.

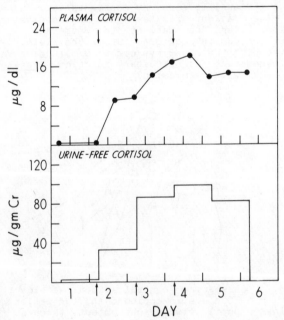

Figure 5.3. Patient with secondary hypoadrenalism was given cortisone acetate im (↓) for three days and plasma cortisol and urine cortisol were determined for several days. Note that steroid levels remain high after the injections are discontinued (normal UC in this lab, < 40 ug/gm creatinine).

When the patient is stable (e.g., no fever, infection, etc.) and can take po meds, then oral hydrocortisone 20 mg tid or cortisone acetate 25 mg bid is given until discharge from the hospital. Maintenance glucocorticoid therapy consists of hydrocortisone 20-30 mg/day in divided doses bid to tid or cortisone acetate 25-37.5 mg/day given bid (before breakfast and evening meal). The adequacy of glucocorticoid replacement can be assessed while taking these meds by measuring urine cortisol (UC). Prednisone 5-7.5 mg/day may be used but UC is not helpful in these cases since prednisone is not measured in this assay.

If the preoperative evaluation demonstrates the patient to be hypothyroid, pituitary surgery need not be postponed. Doses of analgesic medications are reduced to accommodate the decreased metabolism and replacement L-thyroxine is begun, starting at a dose of 25-50 ug/day for 2-3 weeks, increased to 50-100 ug/day for 2-3 weeks and then, maintained at 100-200 ug/day (2 ug/kg body weight/day).

A significant increase in urine output immediately after pituitary surgery usually indicates diabetes insipidus but diabetes mellitus must be excluded. Replacement with intravenous fluid in amounts equivalent to urine output is justified for several hours. Then reduce the iv rate for for 1-2 hrs and check the serum and urine osmolality. A plasma osmolality above 287 mOsm/kg insures volume contraction and excludes volume overload as the cause of the diuresis. Aqueous vasopressin 5 U is given sc. The urine volume should decrease and serum osmolality should increase over next hour when there is diabetes insipidus. One should be aware of the triphasic response of diuresis-antidiuresis-diuresis after pituitary or hypothalmic injury. One to two days postop there is a diuresis that lasts for 3-5 days (probably due to neurohypophyseal trauma), then amelioration for 4-5 days (due to release of stored ADH granules), followed by full-blown diuresis (the sequela of permanent injury). After the diagnosis of diabetes insipidus is firmly established, there are several methods of controlling the polyuria. If the thirst mechanism is intact, as it usually is, then taking vasopressin is a matter of convenience to avoid having to drink excessively and urinate frequently. The most inexpensive form of ADH is pitressin tannate-in-oil (5 U/ml). One ml injection given intramuscularly every 2-4 days costs $1.00-1.50. Patients with hypertension and those who do not like injections may take DDAVP, 0.05-0.15 ml once to twice/day. This medication is absorbed through the nasal mucosa by blowing the solution out of a cannula directed into the nares. Cost is a factor ($0.60-5.00/day). Lysine vasopressin (Diapid) nasal spray is effective but must be used at frequent intervals (every 3 to 6 hours).

Post-operative radiation of the sella is usually prescribed for patients with large tumors since it is rare to completely remove all tumor during surgery. An attempt may be made to wean the patient from maintenance glucocorticoids three to six months postoperatively if there is a good possibility of preserved ACTH function. The following regimen is suggested in a typical patient taking cortisone acetate 25 mg at 7-8 AM and 12.5 mg at 5-6 PM. Withhold the PM steroid for 1-2 weeks, then withhold the Am steroid every other morning for 1-2 weeks. Measure the plasma cortisol prior to the scheduled AM ingestion of the steroid (approximately 48 hrs since last dose). If this value is 5 ug/dl, there is not much chance for successful withdrawal and return to maintenance replacement is recommended. Even if the plasma cortisol is > 5 ug/dl there is no assurance of adequate pituitary-adrenal reserve and some form of dynamic stress testing is necessary, such as insulin-induced hypoglycemia (page7) or a short metyrapone overnight study (page 10). If these are normal, then glucocorticoids are discontinued; if abnormal or borderline, the patient is returned to maintenance doses or a least the use of glucocorticoids during periods of physiological stress. Patients should double or triple their maintenance glucocorticoid dose during these episodes of stress (fever, flu, diarrhea, minor surgery, etc.). Some form of indentification (Medic-Alert) noting the diagnosis of hypopituitarism and steroid dependence should be worn by these patients.

In hypogonadal men, replacement androgen is needed to preserve libido and potency as well as muscle mass and stamina. Testosterone given as testosterone cypionate 200 mg (Depo-Testosterone) or testosterone enanthate 200 mg (Delatestryl) im every 2-4 weeks is the best choice. Intramuscular testosterone has many advantages: it is effective, inexpensive, serum levels are maintained for at least two weeks after injection, and one avoids the complication of cholestatic hepatitis that is seen with oral androgens.

Syndrome of Inappropiate ADH Secretion

Antidiuretic hormone secretion in the presence of low plasma osmolality and in absence of physiologic states that cause ADH secretion (e.g., dehydration, hypovolemia, or hypotension) characterizes the syndrome of inappropiate antidiuretic hormone (SIADH). Continual ADH secretion leads to decrease free water clearance and dilutional hyponatremia. The diagnosis of SIADH should be suspected when there is a combination of hyponatremia (serum sodium usually < 130 meq/l) and an inappropiately concentrated urine. The urine sodium is usually > 20 meq/l in SIADH patients who are taking normal amounts of salt. This is in contrast to patients with hyponatremia with decreased effective blood volume (e.g., heart failure, ascites) where renal tubular resorption of sodium is increased and the urine sodium is < 20 meq/l. There are multiple causes of SIADH: 1) ectopic production of ADH (SIADH was first described in patients with bronchogenic carcinoma which remains the most common cause of this syndrome); 2) central nervous system disorders (head injuries, vascular lesions, infections, Guillain-Barre syndrome, and acute intermittent porphyria); 3) drugs (vincristine, chlorpropamide, carbamazepine); and 4) endocrine disease (Addison's disease, hypothyroidism). The clinical features are weight gain and symptoms of hyponatremia (weakness, lethargy, and mental confusion). Seizures are treated with intravenous hypertonic saline (5%) in amounts to increase the serum sodium to 120 meq/l. All SIADH patients are volume replete and need restriction of fluids to < 1000 ml/day. Sodium loading is not helpful since these patients respond by excreting it into the urine without correcting the hyponatremia. If fluid restriction does not work or the underlying disorder cannot be treated effectively (e.g., oat cell carcinoma of the lung), then administration of demeclocycline 300 mg tid to qid to inhibit ADH's action on the renal tubule may prove effective.

References

Burch W: A survey of results with transsphenoidal surgery in Cushing's disease. N Engl J Med 308:103, 1983.

Clemmons DR, Van Wyk JJ, Ridgway EC et al: Evaluation of acromegaly by radioimmunoassay of somatomedin-C. N Engl J Med 301:1138, 1979.

Frohman LA: Diseases of anterior pituitary, in Felig P, Baxter JD, Broadus AE, Frohman LA (eds): Endocrinology and Metabolism. New York, McGraw-Hill, 1981, 151-231.

Gold EM: The Cushing's syndromes: changing views of diagnosis and treatment. Ann Int Med 90:829, 1979.

Jordan RM, Kendall JW, Kerber CW: The primary empty sella. Amer J Med 62:569, 1977.

Kleinberg DL, Boyd AE III, Wardlaw SW, Frantz AG et al: Pergolide for the treatment of pituitary tumors secreting prolactin or growth hormone. N Engl J Med 309:704, 1983.

Krieger DT: Physiopathology of Cushing's disease. Endocr Rev 4:22, 1983.

Liddle GW: Tests of pituitary adrenal suppressibility in the diagnosis of Cushing's syndrome. J Clin Endocrinol Metab 20:1539, 1960.

Neelon FA, Goree JA, Lebovitz HE: The primary empty sella: clinical and radiographic characteristics and endocrine function. Medicine 52:73, 1973.

Neelon FA, Syndor CF: The assessment of pituitary function. Disease-a-Month 24(4):1-55, 1978.

Robertson GL: Diseases of posterior pituitary, in Felig P, Baxter JD, Broadus AE, Frohman LA (eds): Endocrinology and Metabolism. New York, McGraw-Hill, 1981, pp 251-277.

Schlechte J, Sherman B, Halmi N, et al: Prolactin-secreting pituitary tumors in amenorrheic women: a comprehensive study. Endocrin Rev 1:295, 1980.

Thorner MO: Prolactinoma, in Krieger DT, Bardin CW (eds): Current Therapy in Endocrinology 1983-1984. Burlington, Ontario, BC Decker, 1983, pp 34-38.

Tyrell JB, Brooks RM, Fitzgerald PA, Cofoid PB, Forsham PH, Wilson CB: Cushing's disease: selective transsphenoidal resection of pituitary microadenomas. N Engl J Med 298:753, 1978.

Chapter 6

Amenorrhea

Menstrual dysfunction is frequent in many disorders. The absence of menses is normal prior to puberty, during pregnancy, and after ovarian function ceases (menopause). Amenorrhea, defined as absence of menstruation in any female < 16 yrs of age (primary amenorrhea) or the absence of menses for > 6 months in a woman of child-bearing age with a history of menstruation (secondary amenorrhea), requires evaluation. Normal menstruation depends upon normal anatomy and physiology: 1) patent outlet (normal vagina and cervix); 2) uterus that responds to estrogen and progesterone stimulation; 3) ovaries that respond to gonadotropins with estrogen and progesterone production; and 4) the pituitary and hypothalamus which sense the hormone milieu and respond with release of gonadotropins. The diagnostic workup begins with the history and physical examination in an attempt to segregate the causes of amenorrhea as to the organ abnormality: outlet tract, uterus, ovary, or CNS (pituitary and hypothalamus). Localizing the cause(s) of amenorrhea often presents a challenge.

Age, history, and physical examination give helpful clues as to the etiology. Pubertal age females with amenorrhea are more likely to have outlet abnormalities and ovarian dysgenesis whereas older women who have had prior menses are more likely to have pituitary-hypothalamic disorders as the cause of amenorrhea. A history of weight loss, amenorrhea, bulemia, and bradycardia in an otherwise healthy teenager suggests anorexia nervosa. Postpartum amenorrhea and inability to nurse may be secondary to pituitary hermorrhage (Sheehan's syndrome). Amenorrhea due to destruction of the endometrium (Asherman's syndrome) and scarification as a result of overzealous postpartum curettage should also be considered. Physical examination identifies most causes of primary amenorrhea (listed in order of decreasing frequency): 1) Turner's syndrome (gonadal dysgenesis) with sexual infantilism (absent breast development) and its somatic manifestations (short stature, webbed neck, widely spaced nipples, etc.); 2) congenital absence of vagina with normal growth and sexual development (breast, pubic and axillary hair, feminine figure); 3) testicular feminization with blind vaginal pouch, scant pubic hair, inguinal hernia, and often palpable inguinal masses; and 4) imperforate hymen. Galactorrhea with amenorrhea indicates a pituitary abnormality (possible prolactinoma). Amenorrhea may relate to underlying chronic disease (hepatic and renal failure) or to other endocrine disorders such as thyroid disease (hyperthyroidism and hypothyroidism), adrenal disease (hypocortisolism and hypercortisolism), and hirsutism (page 85).

Workup of Amenorrhea

When the diagnosis is not evident from the history and physical examination and the urine pregnancy test for chorionic gonadotropin is negative, the following studies are performed: 1) serum prolactin to assess whether hyperprolactinemia is the cause of the secondary amenorrhea; 2) serum gonadotropins (FSH and LH) to determine if there is primary ovarian failure; and 3) progestin administration to assess the level of endogenous estrogen and the competence of the outlet tract. Provera, 10 mg po q d for 5 days, is given. Vaginal bleeding should occur within a week after Provera is discontinued. Withdrawal bleeding indicates normal endogenous estrogen levels since proliferative endometrium (which is under estrogenic stimulation) must be present if Provera is to have an effect (progesterone converts proliferative into a secretive endometrium). Withdrawal bleeding will not occur in outlet obstruction (congenital absent vagina), uterine agenesis (testicular feminization, XY gonadal dysgenesis), endometrial scarring (Asherman's syndrome), or in the "unprimed" uterus as in low estrogen states (gonadal failure, hypopituitarism). Patients who have withdrawal bleeding and normal serum prolactin levels have anovulation as the etiology of their amenorrhea (polycystic ovarian disease, extraglandular estrogen formation, psychogenic causes). Patients with elevated prolactin levels need brain CT scan to evaluate for mass lesions of the pituitary (page 61).

An additional study to perform in women who do not have withdrawal bleeding after Provera administration is to prime the endometrium with estrogen (Premarin 1.25 mg bid for 21 days) followed by progesterone (Provera 10 mg q d for 5 days). Withdrawal bleeding will not occur in outlet obstruction or end-organ abnormality (uterine agenesis or Asherman's syndrome). Females with testicular feminization will not have withdrawal bleeding since no uterus is present. These women represent a classic example of hormone resistance, in this case, androgen-resistance. Testicular feminization is inherited as a X-linked recessive trait. The genotype is XY although the phenotype is unmistakenly female. These young women present with primary amenorrhea, normal growth and development, and have well-developed

secondary sex features (breasts and feminine figure). The
skin and its appendages are not stimulated by normal or high
normal levels of serum testosterone leading to little to no
axillary or pubic hair. Testes are present in the inguinal
canal or are within the abdomen. These gonads are removed
because of their incidence of neoplasia approaches 50% in
women > 30 yrs old.

Withdrawal bleeding after therapy with estrogen-
progesterone confirms the presence of a uterus that
responses to hormonal stimulation and localizes the
abnormality to either the ovary or the
pituitary-hypothalmus. The gonadotropins, FSH and LH, are
elevated in gonadal failure. FSH values > 40 mIU/ml are
diagnostic of primary gonadal failure. LH levels are
elevated prior to ovulation and are not as specific for
gonadal failure as raised FSH levels.

FLOW DIAGRAM USED IN THE EVALUATION OF AMENORRHEA

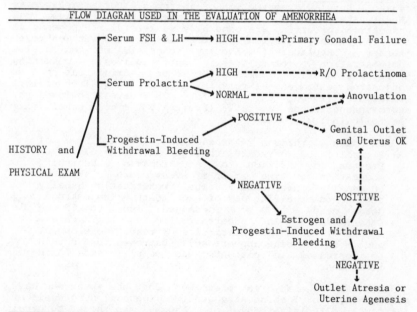

Patients with typical Turner's syndrome have short
stature (adult height rarely above 58 inches); stocky build,
webbed neck, widely spaced nipples ("shield chest"), and
cubitus valgus. These patients usually have the 45,XO
genotype, but mosaicism is not uncommon (XO/XX). Any
hypergonadotropic patient under 35 years old who has primary

amenorrhea needs karyotyping to exclude the presence of Y chromosome since malignant tumors develop in about 25% of these dysgenetic gonads. A patient who has a negative karotype for Y chromosome and does _not_ have the typical features of Turner's syndrome needs a H-Y antigen determination. H-Y antigen is a male-specific cell surface marker and is controlled by a gene found on the short arm of the Y chromosome. Gonadectomy is necessary for those patients with evidence of Y chromosome or H-Y antigen. Premature menopause occurs much earlier than average age of menopause (50 yrs); is associated with elevated FSH and LH levels; and may be due to surgical oophorectomy, autoimmune oophoritis (e.g., associated with polyglandular failure), radiation to the pelvis, or chemotherapy. If the serum LH is < 5 mIU/ml, then hypopituitarism is likely (page 66).

Treatment of the amenorrhea is directed to the specific cause. Surgical correction of anatomic abnormalies such as imperforate hymen, congenital agenesis of vagina, and endometrial scarring are generally successful. Hypogonadism due to primary ovarian failure is treated with estrogen therapy. Replacement therapy consists of the cyclic administration of oral contraceptives containing estrogen-progestin combination or administration of conjugated estrogens (Premarin 1.25-2.5 mg q d) or ethinyl estradiol (20-50 ug/day) for 25 days followed by medroxyprogesterone acetate (Provera). A good schelude is the following:

On days 1 through 24 of each month, take 1.25 mg of Premarin; on days 20 through 24, take 10 mg of Provera in addition to the Premarin. Beginning medication on the first of every month establishes an easily remembered routine. Menstruation usually begins on the 27th day of each month. The estrogen dose needs to be increased (up to 10 mg Premarin/day) in pubertal females to achieve secondary sex characteristics (breast development and more feminine appearance). Estrogen dose should be decreased in patients who complain of fluid retention.

The same therapy is prescibed for the women who have gonadectomy for Y chromosome genotype (gonadal dysgenesis or testicular feminization) or those who have surgical oophorectomy or premature menopause. Secondary hypogonadism is managed as far as the underlying disorder can be corrected (e.g., surgery for a pituitary tumor or bromocriptine for prolactinoma). Chronic anovulation related to polycystic ovarian disease is usually treated with oral contraceptives in an attempt to suppress androgen production (page 88). Other endocrine diseases associated with anovulation (e.g., Cushing's syndrome, Addison's disease, thyrotoxicosis, hypothyroidism) should be treated first. Psychogenic causes of chronic anovulation include anorexia nervosa and amenorrhea of emotional stress. Treatment is directed to the primary cause in these patients and estrogen replacement is not prescibed.

References

Griffin JE, Edwards C, Madden JD, Harrod MJ, Wilson JD: Congenital absence of the vagina. Ann Intern Med 85:224, 1976.

Klein SM, Garcia CR: Asherman's syndrome: a critique and current review. Fertil Steril 24:722, 1973.

Moghissi KS, Syner FN, Evans TN: A composite picture of the menstrual cycle. Am J Obstet Gynecol 114:405, 1972.

Ohno S: The role of H-Y antigen in primary sex determination. JAMA 239:217, 1978.

Speroff L, Glass R, Kase NG: Amenorrhea, in Clinical Gynecologic Endocrinology and Infertility 2nd ed., Baltimore, Williams & Wilkins, 1978, pp 93-121.

Chapter 7

Impotence

Impotence is the inability to achieve or to maintain a penile erection which will allow the patient to engage in coitus. Recurrent or persistent impotence (as opposed to occasional episodes of "honeymoon" impotence) is a considerable problem. Impotence increases with age so that approximately 20% of the males at age 60 yrs and 50% of males age 70 yrs are impotent.

Potency is affected by libido and physical health. Libido, the physiologic and mental drive for sexual satisfaction, is essential for potency. Libido varies among individuals and within each individual is influenced by social and sexual experiences, by physical and mental illness, and by medication. Libido tends to decrease with age but loss of sexual interest and drive is most commonly situational. Men may experience dissatifaction with their accomplishments, frustration, fatigue from overwork, or discouragement and a lack of communication with their sexual partner. These factors as well as depression and neurosis account for most impotence in younger men, so-called psychogenic or functional impotence. Drugs that diminish libido include alcohol, tranquilizers, sedatives, opiates, antihypertensives, and estrogens. Hypogonadism affects libido and is discussed below.

Potency depends on normal anatomy and physiologic function. The erectile mechanism requires intact neurologic, vascular, and endocrine systems. Impairment of any one of these can produce impotence.

Neurogenic impotence: Any disruption of the parasympathetic autonomous nervous system impairs erectile ability. Stimulation of the S2-S4 nerve roots via the nervi erigentes causes relaxation of specialized vascular smooth muscles ("polsters") leading to engorgement of the corpora cavernosa. Many diseases interfere with parasympathetic outflow: diabetes mellitus, alcoholism, heavy metal intoxication, cord tumors, and multiple sclerosis. Surgical procedures such as perineal prostatectomy or retroperineal dissection also may impair the erectile mechanism.

Vascular impotence: Full erection requires adequate penile blood flow. Obstruction of the aorta, iliac vessels, hypogastric, or pudendal arteries can lead to impotence. An example is Leriche's syndrome of lower extremity claudication and impotence. Small arteriole disease associated with diabetes mellitus also causes impotence.

Anatomic impotence: Genitourinary conditions such as Peyronie's disease, urethritis, severe chordee, and penile trauma may result in impotence.

Endocrine impotence: The hormonal milieu must be adequate for potency. Normal adrenal and thyroid function are important to male sexual function, but the testosterone production is paramount. Testosterone stimulates protein synthesis (muscle mass) and virilization (enlargement of the phallus, scrotal rugosity and pigmentation, and hair growth on face, chest, and back). High intratesticular levels of testosterone are essential to normal spermatogenesis. Testosterone also affects the limbic system and is probably one of the factors responsible for aggressive behavior that is considered normally masculine. In the skin (hair follicles and sweat glands) and in the prostate gland, testosterone is reduced by 5-alpha-reductase to dihydrotestosterone which is the metabolically active form of the hormone in these tissues. Testosterone deficiency (hypogonadism) is an important cause of endocrine impotence and is most amenable to treatment.

Workup of the Impotent Patient

The history is important. The patient who can sometimes have normal erections and yet be impotent at other times most likely has functional or psychogenic impotence. Normal erections imply that the neurogenic, vascular, and endocrine systems are intact. Ask about early morning penile erections. Does the patient have multiple sex partners? Are there identifiable stress factors? If the patient has diabetes mellitus, are there other symptoms of peripheral or autonomic neuropathy? Is there claudication which might explain incomplete penile tumescence? What is the patient's age and when did impotence develop? Failure to virilize by the mid-to-late teens implies pituitary or gonadal abnormality which must be thoroughly investigated. Are there other endocrine dysfunction in the past to suggest polyglandular failure? What medications is the patient taking?

The physical examination may give clues about hypogonadism. What is the testicular size? Normal testes are 4.5±1.0 cm long and 2.5±0.5 cm wide. Are the testes pea size and firm as is typical of Klinefelter's syndrome? Klinefelter's syndrome (primary testicular failure due to chromatin-positive gonadal dysgenesis) is a common cause of hypogonadism that affects 1 out of 500 males. Many of these patients develop secondary sex characteristics during puberty since the Leydig cells have not yet involuted. The skin of the chronic hypogonadal male is smooth and soft with crows-foot wrinkles about the eyes and mouth. Anosmia suggests hypogonadotropic hypogonadalism (Kallman's syndrome)? Is there evidence for pituitary disease? Physical findings of chronic disease such as hepatic or renal failure and other endocrine diseases such as hypoadrenalism, acromegaly, and hypothyroidism should be sought as potential causes of impotence. In the diabetic with impotence, signs of peripheral neuropathy (absent ankle jerks, decreased vibratory sensation) are usually present.

Laboratory studies: Serum testosterone should be measured in each impotent patient. Normal adult values range from 300-1200 ng/dl. There is some diurnal variation in the serum testosterone; the highest levels occurring between 6 and 9 AM with a 15-40% decrement by late afternoon. The lower values are still well within the normal range so a single determination is sufficient for diagnostic purposes. Testosterone production decreases with age and serum testosterone levels are slightly decreased but remain well within the normal range. Since testosterone production is controlled by luteinizing hormone (LH), any disturbance of the hypothalamic-pituitary-testicular axis may lead to testosterone deficiency and impotency. In normal men there is no relationship between the level of serum LH (range 4-24 mIU/ml) and the serum testosterone (range 300-1200 ng/dl). However in primary testicular disease the serum LH is very helpful since it is elevated in the absence of the negative feedback of testosterone. Thus, patients with primary hypogonadism will have low serum testosterone levels and high serum LH levels. Secondary hypogonadism is often due to a prolactinoma which usually presents late (macroadenoma) with impotence being the predominant clinical symptom. Serum prolactin should be ordered if anything suggests hypogonadism in the middle and late age male. Occasionally patients with hyperthyroidism present with impotence but the serum testosterone is elevated (> 1200 ng/ml) because hyperthyroidism increases the sex hormone binding globulin (the free testosterone concentration is normal). Treatment of the hyperthyroidism will usually correct the impotence.

The most common cause of <u>organic impotence is diabetes mellitus.</u> This is usually due to a combination of vascular obstruction as result of arteriosclerosis and autonomic neuropathy. An occasional diabetic may have primary testicular failure which produces impotence. Because hypogonadism is treatable, one should measure the level of serum testosterone.

In summary, determination of serum testosterone, serum LH, and serum prolactin will usually detect any endocrine cause of impotence.

<u>Etiology of Hypogonadism:</u> Primary hypogonadism may be caused by a variety of disorders. Idiopathic testicular failure, sometimes associated with polyglandular endocrine failure, is the most common. Gonadal dysgenesis, testicular torsion, and trauma are other causes. Secondary hypogonadism may be due to constitutional delay of growth and development in the adolescent, to isolated hypogonadotropic hypogonadism, or to any of the causes of hypo-pituitarism (page 66). Other endocrine causes such as acromegaly and Addison's disease should be managed prior to any treatment of associated hypogonadism.

<u>Treatment of Hypogonadism:</u> Testosterone replacement is simple, effective, and safe. Esterified derivatives of testosterone are given intramuscularly assuring constant levels necessary to maintain muscle mass, beard growth, and libido. <u>Testosterone cypionate or testosterone enanthate 200 mg im every 2-4 weeks</u> restores potency in most hypogonadal males. Replacement is continued indefinitely. Lower doses (50-100 mg im q 2-3 weeks) are used in the adolescent hypogonadal male in order to avoid excessive stimulation of epiphyseal cartilage growth and maturation. Excessive androgen accelerates the maturation leading to bone closure and short stature. Orally administrated alkylated testosterone derivatives are <u>not</u> used because their effects on potency are not predictable and there are risks of hepatotoxicity with long-term therapy. If the patient is not hypogonadal yet still has organic impotence (e.g., diabetes mellitus), mechanical devices such as an inflatable prosthesis provide a treatment of impotence.

<u>Functional or Psychogenic Impotence:</u> The prevalence of impotence vastly exceeds that of all endocrine disorders. Therefore, most instances of sexual dysfunction are not related to a primary endocrine problem. Probably the most accurate means of distinquishing psychogenic from other causes of impotence is to monitor nocturnal penile tumescence (diminished or absent in most organic impotence). Androgen treatment of patients with functional impotence is not helpful. Several studies have shown that the effect of

testosterone in these patients matches that of placebo therapy alone. Chronic testosterone treatment of eugonadal males decreases sperm count and testicular volume so this is not even a good placebo drug. Appropiate evaluation and counseling as to the pathophysiology of impotence and to the factors that affect libido are necessary in treating these patients.

References

Burch WM: Impotence. Consultant 22:275, 1982.

Karacan I: Diagnosis of erectile impotence in diabetes mellitus. An objective and specific method. Ann Intern Med 92:334, 1980.

Smith KD: Testicular function in the aging male, in DeGroot LJ (ed): Endocrinology. New York, Grune & Stratton, 1979, pp 1577-1581.

Spark RF, White RA, Connolly PB: Impotence is not always psychogenic. Newer insights into hypothalamic-pituitary-gonadal dysfunction. JAMA 243:750, 1980.

Schwartz MF, Kolodny RC, Masters WH: Plasma testosterone levels of sexually functional and dysfunctional men. Arch Sex Behav 9:355, 1980.

Chapter 8

Hirsutism

Women often complain of extra hair and seek advice on how the manage this cosmetic problem. Hirsutism refers to excessive hair growth in the androgen-responsive skin zones typically considered to be masculine in distribution. Terminal (coarse) hairs develop on the upper lip, sideburns, chin, neck, chest, lower abdomen (male escutcheon), and perineum. The degree of hair stimulation varies depending on _race_ (Orientals, American Indians, and Negroes have less hirsutism than Caucasians), _genetic background_ (those of Mediterranean origin are typically more hirsute than those of Nordic origin), and _family history._ Darkly-pigmented Caucausian women tend to be more hirsute than light complected females. The incidence of hirsutism increases after menopause. Since our culture epitomizes virtually hairless women (e.g., models found on magazine covers), some women complain of relatively mild hirsutism not realizing the range of normal variation and the significance of factors mentioned above.

The cause of true hirsutism is hyperandrogenism in more than 90% of patients. The primary androgen that stimulates the hair follicle is testosterone. The testosterone production rate is increased in nearly all hirsute women although the serum or plasma testosterone may be in the upper range of normal. Serum testosterone levels are only indirect determinations of androgen activity. The free or unbound testosterone, the bioactive moiety, constitutes less than 1-3 % of the total serum testosterone, the remainder being bound to sex hormone-binding globulin (SHBG). Hyperandrogenemia itself decreases the concentration of SHBG so that the total serum testosterone is not a true reflection of androgen status.

Testosterone is produced from three sources in the normal female: ovary (25% of the total), adrenal (25% of the total), and peripheral tissues (50% of the total). The peripheral tissues (fat, muscle) convert weak androgens (primarily androstenedione) secreted by the adrenal and ovary into testosterone. In evaluating the hirsute female one tries to identify the source of the hyperandrogenemia: ovary, adrenal, or both.

In evaluating the hirsute patient we need to know several historical points:

Age of onset: Was it prior to the onset of menstruation? Was pubic and axillary hair growth associated with hirsutism? (Hirsutism before age 9 suggests an adrenal source such as congenital adrenal hyperplasia.) Did hair growth start soon after menarche? Progress slowly since menarche? (If yes, then history is typical of either polycystic ovary disease (PCOD) or idiopathic hirsutism.) Did the hirsutism start at menopause or later? (If it starts several years after menopause, beware of androgen-secreting tumor of the ovary or the adrenal gland.)
Mode of onset: Did the hirsutism develop gradually or an abrupt onset? (Abrupt or recent onset suggest significant pathology, i.e., an androgen-secreting tumor.)
Menstrual abnormalities: Are menses regular? If so, then significant ovarian or adrenal pathology is unlikely. Menstrual abnormalities with chronic anovulation is the rule in severe PCOD. Although hirsutism is rare in hyperprolactinemic states, a history of galactorrhea should be sought.
Medications: Is the patient taking meds that are known to promote hirsutism? Androgens, dilantin, diazoxide, and minoxidil are known to do this is varying degrees.
Family history: Is there a family history of chronic ovulatory problems? Any wedge resections of ovaries for PCOD?   PCOD appears to be inherited as an autosomal dominant trait and the family history is positive in 40% of cases with PCOD.

The physical examination should tell whether the patient is simply hirsute or whether virilization is present. The virilized patient is not only severely hirsute but also has clitoromegaly, frontal or occipital balding, deepening of voice, enlargement of thyroid cartilage (Adam's apple), and increased muscle mass. Breast atrophy and loss of body contours occur with severe virilization. Virilization outside the neonatal period suggests a tumor of the ovary or adrenal although severe PCOD may sometimes cause virilization. Physical stigmata of Cushing's syndrome should be sought. The pelvic exam is particularly important in assessing perineal hair distribution, clitoromegaly, uterus, and adnexal masses. Obese females may need ultrasonography to determine ovarian size.

The following laboratory studies are needed to evaluate hirsutism: serum testosterone, free testosterone (if available), serum dehydroepiandosterone sulfate (DHEA-S), and serum LH and FSH. If Cushing's syndrome cannot be excluded clinically, a 24-hr urine cortisol or an overnight dexamethasone study is done (page 12). A 24 hr urine for

17-ketosteroids reflects the serum DHEA-S concentrations and evaluates adrenal androgen output. 17-Ketosteroids do not measure testosterone. 17-Ketosteroids alone are rarely sufficient to evaluate hyperandrogenic syndromes. Because of the pulsatile secretion of FSH and LH from the pituitary, three blood samples should be drawn at 30 minutes intervals and these 3 samples pooled for determination of LH and FSH levels. Dynamic studies such as dexamethasone suppression studies and gonadotropin stimulatory studies do not help distinguish whether the androgen source is the adrenal or ovary and are generally avoided.

The source of the hyperandrogenemia can often be identified on the basis of the history, physical exam, and these laboratory studies. Therapy can be directed to the specific cause of the hirsutism. Androgen-secreting tumors are associated with serum testosterone > 200 ng/dl or DHEA-S > 4000 ng/ml, rapidly progressing hirsutism with virilization, and an onset usually much later than menarche. The ovary is the usual site of testosterone-producing tumors (arrhenoblastoma, Sertoli-Leydig cell tumor, etc.) and the adrenal, the site for carcinomas that produce excessive DHEA-S and urinary 17-KS. Localization of the androgen-secreting tumor with computerized tomography is recommended since an occasional adrenal tumor may secrete only testosterone and be missed if surgery is prematurely directed to the ovaries. If there is galactorrhea/ prolactinemia, the hyperandrogenism is part of the amenorrhea-galactorrhea syndrome associated with PCOD and overproduction of adrenal androgens. The mechanism of hyperandrogenism in this syndrome is not understood. Treatment of the hyperprolactinemia with bromocryptine (or surgical removal of the prolactinoma) will often help the hirsutism. Drug-related hirsutism is diagnosed by the history.

Most of the women who present with hirsutism do not have any ominous cause but rather fit into a spectrum of syndromes associated with normal or modestly elevated serum testosterones and elevated free testosterone. All of these are associated with varying degrees of ovarian stromal hyperplasia. Polycystic ovary disease is by far the most common variant. PCOD has its onset just after menarche, and is characterized by chronic anovulation (amenorrhea/ oligomenorrhea and dysfunctional uterine bleeding), and slowly progressive hirsutism. A familial tendency may be noted for similar problems. Many, but not all, of the patients are obese, and some women have no hirsutism but present for evaluation of infertility. Enlarged ovaries are palpable in about 1/2 the subjects. The ratio of LH to FSH is often elevated (> 2.5).

There is a self-perpetuating cycle of hormonal events associated with polycystic ovaries. Increased ovarian production of testosterone blocks follicule maturation leading to numerous follicles in varying stages of development. These follicles have limited growth potential and undergo atresia, leading to an increase in the stromal compartment. The stroma normally secretes significant amounts of testosterone and androstenedione and its increased mass results in secretion of a greater amount of androgen. Peripheral conversion of androstenedione into estrone sensitizes the pituitary gonadotrope (as normally happens with increased estrogen levels prior to mid-cycle LH surge) to respond to GnRH leading to LH production. LH stimulates the ovarian stroma to produce more testosterone (which stimulates hair growth and blocks follicular maturation leading to atresia, etc.) and androstendione (which is converted to estrone and leads to more LH production, etc.). What triggers the cycle is unknown.

Treatment of PCOD is directed at suppression of ovarian production of androgens using oral contraceptive agents. Ortho-Novum 2 mg and Demulen have had wide use for treating PCOD. Ortho-Novum 2 mg is started on 5th day of menses, given for 21 days and repeated cyclically. After 2-3 months of treatment androgens levels are remeasured. If these results are normal or there has been > 50% reduction, treatment is continued realizing that any amelioration of the hirsutism will be gradual with a maximal therapeutic effect after 9-12 months. The usual precautions related to oral contraceptives (blood pressure, venous thrombosis, etc.) are necessary. Clomiphene may be used to induce ovulation in those patients who desire pregnancy. Ovarian wedge resection may be used for patients who fail to ovulate with clomiphene.

A few hirsute women with normal size ovaries and normal LH/FSH ratios will have elevated DHEA-S without evidence of Cushing's syndrome or androgen-producing adrenal tumor. The hyperandrogenism is thought to be ACTH dependent. Some of these females have a partial defect in adrenal 17-hydroxylase which leads to raised 17-hydroxyprogesterone (17OHP) levels in the serum. These patients are diagnosed by a provocative ACTH study. Baseline 17OHP is drawn and Cortrosyn 0.25 mg is given im and 17-OHP measured 1 hr later. Patients with a partial enzymatic defect demonstrate a 5-10 fold rise in 17OHP levels (normal < twofold). Treatment consists of dexamethasone 0.5 mg hs (or prednisone 5 mg hs). If, after a month's therapy, the DHEA-S level is above 1000 ng/ml, oral contraceptives are added to the regimen. Any pituitary-adrenal suppressive treatment must be weighed in regards to benefits (lessening of hirsutism) versus side effects (taking glucocorticoid blocks the normal cortisol response that occurs in stress situations, and a Cushingoid state develops if excessive glucocorticoids are taken).

Some hirsute females have normal menses and normal serum androgens. These women have idiopathic hirsutism probably due to increased sensitivity of the hair follicle to normal circulating amounts of androgens. Treatment with oral contraceptives helps these patients since serum testosterone falls with ovarian suppression. In addition, since estrogens increase SHBG the level of free testosterone is even lower. The antiandrogen drug, cyproterone acetate, appears to be the most effective medication for idiopathic hirsutism but is not approved for use in the United States. Spironolactone and cimetidine have antiandrogen activity but are generally much less effective than oral contraceptives.

Medical therapy can at times decrease the rate of hair growth and reduce the texture of the hair in the androgen-sensitive areas. Other cosmetic measures are important to reduce the hirsutism. Techniques to remove the unwanted hair include bleaching, tweezing, hot wax epilation, chemical depilatories, shaving, and electrolysis. Shaving is the safest way to remove hair and has the least untoward reactions. Patients should be informed that shaving does not increase hair growth or increase the thickness of the hair shaft. The only permanent means to remove the hair is to ablate the hair follicle. Electrolysis or short-wave radio-frequency thermolysis is effective but requires the skill of an experienced electrologist and is expensive. The combination of medical therapy, frequent shaving, judicious electrolysis, and a sympathetic physician are necessary to successfully manage this common medical problem.

References

Givens JR: Hirsutism and hyperandrogenism. Adv Intern Med 21: 221, 1976.

Givens JR: Hirsutism, in Krieger DT, Bardin CW (eds): Current Therapy in Endocrinology 1983-1984. Burlington, Ontario, BC Decker, 1983, pp 143-146.

Kirschner MA: Polycystic and sclerocystic ovaries, in Krieger DT, Bardin CW (eds): Current Therapy in Endocrinology 1983-1984. Burlington, Ontario, BC Decker, 1983, pp 404-409.

Mauvais-Jarv P, Kuttenn F, Mowszowicz I: Hirsutism. Monographs on Endocrinology. Berlin, Springer-Verlag, 1981.

Yen SSC: The polycystic ovary syndrome. Clin Endocrinol 12:177, 1980.

Chapter 9

Gynecomastia

Gynecomastia (male breast hypertrophy) is a frequent clinical problem since most males have breast enlargement sometime during their life. Breast development is the same for males and females until puberty when estrogen levels rise dramatically in females. Estrogen is the primary hormone that stimulates both ductal and stromal breast development. Understanding of estrogen metabolism in men is important in assessing the causes of gynecomastia. Estradiol, a potent estrogen, stimulates breast enlargement in both sexes. Aromatization of testosterone's A ring accounts for most of the estradiol produced in men and occurs primarily in fat tissue. About 10% of serum estradiol comes from its direct secretion from the testes. The fraction of testicular estradiol secretion increases upon gonadotropin (LH) administration. Estrone is another estrogen produced by the peripheral aromatization of androstenedione, an androgen secreted primarily by the adrenal. The levels of estrogen circulating in the adult male are about 200 times lower than serum testosterone levels, yet a perturbation of the ratio of androgen to estrogen by increased estrogen production or decreased testosterone production explains most causes of gynecomastia.

Gynecomastia may be a normal physiologic event, a response to drugs and medications, or a harbinger of disease. Gynecomastia can be unilateral and have no other explanation other than the causes of bilateral breast development. However, care must be taken not to miss the unusual lesions such as breast carcinoma, neurofibroma, hemangioma, and lipoma which all have a different texture on palpation than the finely nodular texture of glandular breast tissue.

Gynecomastia as a physiologic event: There are three stages of life (neonatal, pubertal, and senescent) that gynecomastia relates to normal development. Neonatal gynecomastia is a transient phenomenon, occurs in response to maternal estrogens, and resolves usually within a few weeks of birth. Pubertal gynecomastia occurs in up to 70% of boys and is probably related to increased testicular production of estradiol. Levels of estradiol peak before adult levels of testosterone are obtained that lead to a temporary alteration of the androgen/estrogen ratio. In most boys pubertal gynecomastia disappears within two to three years. Large amounts of breast tissue, described as Tanner stage III or greater (glandular tissue which extends past the areola associated with enlargement and darkening of the areola), that persists beyond the age of 16-17 yrs seldom regress. These young men with persistent pubertal gynecomastia require surgical removal of the glandular tissue. Senescent gynecomastia found in the seventh and eighth decades of life is a diagnosis of exclusion since there are many causes of gynecomastia (e.g., drugs or underlying disease) in this age group. Slightly decreased testosterone levels and increased peripheral aromatization of testosterone to estradiol produces an altered androgen/estrogen ratio causes the gynecomastia in these men.

Drug-related gynecomastia: Drugs cause gynecomastia by many mechanisms. Inhibitors of testosterone synthesis include spironolactone and chemotherapeutic drugs (cyclophosphamide, melphalan, etc.). Cimetidine and spironolactone inhibit testosterone action at the receptor level. Any medication which increases estrogen levels or its effect may lead to gynecomastia. Testosterone therapy itself can cause gynecomastia by peripheral conversion to estradiol. Digitalis and digitoxin are weak estrogen agonists. Diethylstilbestrol therapy used to treat prostatic carcinoma causes gynecomastia which can be prevented with pretreatment irradiation to the breasts (900-1500 rads over 3 days). Treatment with gonadotropins (HCG) increases testicular production of estrogens. Other anecdotal associations of drug-related gynecomastia include digoxin, methyldopa, reserpine, isoniazid, ethionamide, tricyclic antidepressants, phenothiazines, diazepam, hydroxyzine, heroin, and marijuana.

Gynecomastia related to underlying disorder or disease: Hypogonadism as a result of decreased testosterone production or a decrease in its action may cause gynecomastia. Primary testicular failure related to Klinefelter's syndrome (incidence of about 0.2% in the male population) is common and is frequently associated with gynecomastia. Other causes of testicular failure (e.g. anorchism, trauma, orchitis) may be associated with gynecomastia. Gynecomastia found in androgen resistance syndromes such as perineoscrotal hypospadias (Reifenstein's syndrome) is caused by testosterone's decreased effect on typically androgen-sensitive tissues and by increased LH stimulation of testicular estradiol secretion leading to an altered ratio of effective androgen to estrogen.

Increased estrogen production caused by feminizing tumors of the adrenal gland and Leydig cell tumors of the testes is rare. The production of estrogen can be a direct release of estradiol from the tumor or, as in the case of adrenal tumors, an increase in precursor substrate concentration (androstenedione) which is converted to estrogen peripherally. Tumors most likely to cause gynecomastia are gonadotropin (HCG) secreting tumors such as oat cell lung carcinoma, choriocarcinoma, and hepatoblastoma. Testicular aromatase activity is enhanced by HCG leading to increased estradiol secretion.

Certain metabolic and chronic diseases are associated with gynecomastia. Increased substrate for the aromatase enzyme is a common cause for raised estrogen levels. Hyperthyroidism is associated with increased production of adrenal steroids including androstenedione leading to peripheral estrone production and gynecomastia. The metabolism and removal of androstenedione is impaired in chronic liver disease again leading to increase substrate for the aromatase enzyme. Hyperprolactinemia per se does not cause gynecomastia but an elevated prolactin does inhibit LH release leading to lower serum testosterone levels which changes the androgen/estrogen ratio. Refeeding gynecomastia occurs in debilitated patients recovering from starvation and serious systemic illness such as uremia and heart failure.

Workup of Gynecomastia

The history and physical exam identifies most of the causes of gynecomastia. Particular attention to drug and medication history is necessary. Age of the patient is important as it relates to physiological causes of gynecomastia. A history of impotence suggests hypogonadism (page 81). The physical exam should be complete and focus on the breast and testes. In the obese male one often has difficulty distinguishing adipose tissue from glandular tissue. A good method to determine whether breast tissue is present is to place the pulp of the index finger directly over the nipple and apply pressure. One encounters no resistance and easily palpates the underlying rib and intercostal space in the normal and obese male. This area is obscured by glandular tissue in patients with gynecomastia. If there is unilateral breast enlargement, one should take care to examine for signs of cancer (firmness and fixation to skin and surrounding fascia as well as enlarged axillary nodes). The testes are examined for masses. Testicular size and consistency should be recorded (page 82). Is there hepatomegaly? Are there skin signs of hyperestrogenism (e.g. spider angioma)? Is there a goiter or tachycardia to suggest hyperthyroidism?

The laboratory studies ordered are cued from the history and physical examination. The adolescent male with persistent pubertal gynecomastia rarely needs any studies if there is good health, normal growth and development, and a normal genital exam. Klinefelter's syndrome (small firm testes) should be confirmed by a buccal smear looking for sex chromatin (XXY). Serum determinations of testosterone, LH, and prolactin are obtained particularly when there is a history of impotence. Serum HCG (not urine for pregnancy test) and chest X-ray are necessary to exclude tumor-related gynecomastia. Liver function is assessed. Other endocrine studies include urinary 17-ketosteroids to exclude a feminizing adrenal tumor and T4(RIA) and T3U to exclude hyperthyroidism. Even with measurement of serum estradiol and these other studies, the cause for the gynecomastia may not be found.

Treatment of gynecomastia relates to the cause. Discontinuation of the offending medication is often associated with regression of minor degrees of gynecomastia. When the breast is large, it is very rare for the breast to regress even after the cause is removed. Reduction mammoplasty the only effective therapy for these patients. Young men with persistent pubertal gynecomastia need surgical excision since the personal and psychological problems these males encounter are real and cosmetic reduction preserving the areola is beneficial.

References

Brody SA, Loriaux DL: Gynecomastia, in Krieger DT, Bardin CW (eds): Current Therapy in Endocrinology 1983-1984. Burlington, Ontario, BC Decker, 1983, pp 388-391.

Carlson HE: Gynecomastia. N Engl J Med 303:795, 1980.

Treves N: Gynecomastia. Cancer 11:1083, 1958.

Wilson JD, Aiman J, MacDonald PC: The pathogenesis of gynecomastia. Adv Intern Med 25:1, 1980.

Chapter 10

Thyroid Disease

THYROID NODULES

The nodular thyroid gland is a common and important clinical problem. Public awareness that nodules are related to cancer has heightened the anxiety related to this diagnosis. Thyroid nodules can be found in up to 5% of the female population, yet the yearly number of new cases of thyroid cancer is only 0.004% (39/million). Therein lies the difficulty. The risk is real but the chances are small that any given patient will have cancer. To remove every nodular thyroid would submit numerous patients to surgery, most of whom have a benign and mostly asymptomatic disorder. Fortunately, it is possible to identify factors which increase the likelihood that a nodule represents cancer of the thyroid. These risk factors are: <u>age; sex; history of neck irradiation; family history of thyroid carcinoma; and certain physical charactistics of the thyroid itself.</u>

<u>Age:</u> Thyroid nodules are rare in children but about half of them are malignant. There is often a history of radiation exposure. Therefore nodules found in patients under 16 yrs of age should be excised.

<u>Sex:</u> Thyroid nodules are five times more common in females than males. Thyroid cancer is also more frequent in females but only by a factor of two. Therefore there is a greater risk that a male with a thyroid nodule has cancer than that a female has.

<u>History of Irradiation:</u> Irradiation of the head and neck (50-700 rads) is associated with an increased risk of thyroid cancer. The period of latency ranges from 5-35 years with the average around 20 yrs post exposure. Nodules should be removed in patients with this history.

<u>History of familial thyroid carcinoma:</u> Medullary thyroid carcinoma (sometimes associated with hyperparathyroidism and pheochromocytoma as multiple endocrine adenomatosis type II) is often familial. A history for this should be sought. A positive family history is an indication for determination of plasma

calcitonin concentration; an elevated value confirms the
diagnosis.

Physical characteristics of the thyroid gland: The
single nodule is much more likely to be malignant than
the multinodular gland.   The recent onset of a rapidly
enlarging, firm neck mass (especially with associated
hoarseness) is suggestive of infiltrative malignant
disease.   A thyroid mass presenting as a single palpable
nodule (or as part of a multinodular gland) that is very
firm, irregular, or adherent to overlying muscle
generally needs surgical excision.   Carcinomatous
thyroid cells do not trap radionuclides as well as
normal thyroid cells, leading to hypofunctioning, "cold
areas", on thyroid scan.   Hyperfunctioning or "hot"
nodules are very, very unlikely to be malignant.
However, even most "cold" nodules are not malignant and
thus hypofunction of the nodule is not itself very
helpful in making the decision to recommend surgery.
Cysts of the thyroid represent approximately 20% of
"cold" thyroid nodules.   These can be identified by
ultrasound studies.   Simple cysts are rarely malignant
and can be treated with aspiration.   The cyst fluid
should be sent for cytological examination since cystic
degeneration within large neoplastic lesions does occur.
Positive or suspicious cytology requires surgical
removal of the cyst.

Although these factors help to select high risk patients,
only examination of tissue from the nodule is definite.   In
this regard fine needle aspiration helps immensely in the
diagnosis and management of the solitary thyroid nodule.
The critical absolutely essential factor in needle
aspiration is the availability of a cytopathologist who is
expert in interpreting thyroid pathology.   Surgical removal
of all the high risks nodule leads to many patients having
surgery for benign disease.   Fine needle aspiration of these
nodules is safe and offers a rational approach to managing
the thyroid nodule.   I use the following technique of needle
aspiration since small nodules can be well-localized and
fixed between the fingers to allow adequate sampling of
thyroid tissue:

Thyroid masses are best palpated with the patient
sitting or standing.   The physician stands behind the
patient who sits upright in a chair.   The area over the
nodule is prepared with a local antiseptic.   No local
anesthetic is used.   The nodule is fixed between the
index and third finger.   Having the patient swallow
water will help center the nodule between these fingers
as demonstrated in figure 10.1 A.   A 20-21 gauge needle
is affixed to a plastic connecting tube (Venotube;

Abbott Labs) which is attached to a 20-30 ml syringe. The hub of the needle is held between the thumb and index finger of the other hand (fig. 10.1 B). The needle is quickly inserted into the center of the mass. An assistant aspirates the obturator of the syringe to the 10-15 ml mark (fig. 10.1 C).

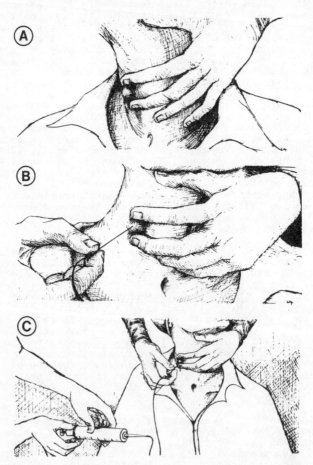

Figure 10.1   Method of Fine Needle Aspiration Biopsy. (A) The patient is seated in a chair and the nodule is localized. (B) Needle is inserted into the nodule. (C) An assistant aspirates the syringe.

If fluid is obtained, the nodule can be massage as the fluid is being aspirated. Any fluid is sent for cytology in a heparinized tube (green stoppered Vacutainer works well) on ice. If no fluid is obtained, the tube is disconnected from the syringe and then the needle removed from the nodule. Any scant material is forced by air onto a glass slide and fixed as any other cytological material (70% ethanol works well). Multiple passes can be made to assure adequacy of the sample. The needle may be washed free of cells with normal saline into a heparinized tube and sent to cytopathology on ice. There the cells can be washed with increasing concentrations of ethanol which lyses red blood cells, filtered through a Millipore filter, and then stained for interpretation by the cytopathologist.

Workup and Management of the Thyroid Nodule

The following should be performed in all patients with thyroid nodule(s): 1) history and physical exam with special attention the neck palpating for lymph nodes and the physical characteristics of the thyroid gland; 2) determination of the serum T4(RIA), T3U, thyroid antimicrosomal antibodies, and occasionally T3(RIA); and 3) thyroid scintiscan (page 6) is generally obtained to determine if the mass is functioning.

If there is clinical evidence of malignancy such as a child with a single firm thyroid nodule or if there is a history of radiation exposure, surgical removal is recommended. Otherwise fine needle aspiration is routinely performed. Although many would recommend ultrasound to determine whether the nodule is cystic or solid, this procedure adds nothing that needle aspiration doesn't contribute.

If the aspiration cytology is suspicious or positive for malignancy, then surgery is recommended. If the cytologic diagnosis is follicular adenoma, surgery is also advised since the cytopathologist often cannot differentiate follicular adenoma from follicular carcinoma. Management for all other cytologic diagnoses (e.g., colloid nodule, hemorrhagic cyst, etc.) depends on the functional characteristics of the nodule. One may be reasonable sure of the benign nature of a thyroid lesion in the following circumstances: 1) The sudden development of a thyroid nodule associated with pain for 4-5 days; this usually represents hemorrhage into a cyst or adenoma. Aspiration will confirmed the diagnosis. 2) Very high titers of antimicrosomal antibodies and a non-diagnostic needle aspiration biopsy indicate a nodular form of Hashimoto's thyroiditis. The TSH may or may not be elevated. 3)

Multinodular goiter with patchy uptake on thyroid scan; if there is an area of unusual firmness, fine needle aspiration is performed. 4) If the nodule is "hot" on scan and the rest of the gland is suppressed.

Thyroid suppressive therapy: Most nodules of the thyroid, including thyroid carcinoma, are responsive to TSH. The goal is to reduce endogenous TSH secretion yet maintain the euthyroid status of these patients by treatment with L-thyroxine 0.15-0.3 mg/day. The dose is determined by assessing the serum T4(RIA) and T3U after a month therapy to insure the FT4 Index (page 4) is higher than the patient's baseline FT4 Index prior to treatment. The response to TRH should be blunted (page 5) and is a sensitive indicator of thyroidal suppression. If there is a rise in serum TSH after TRH, then a larger dose of L-thyroxine is prescribed (e.g., increased from 0.15 mg to 0.2 mg/day). Thyroid suppression is continued for three to six months. If there is > 50% decrease in the thyroid nodule or the nodule disappears, thyroid suppression is continued indefinitely. If there has been < 50% decrease in size, the nodule is reaspirated to see if the original findings can be reproduced. If the cytology is unchanged, thyroid suppression is continued and the patient reevaluated in another six months. If the cytology is suspicious or is consistant with malignancy, surgical removal is indicated. If any thyroid nodule grows in the face of adequate thyroid suppression (with exception of hemorrhage into a cyst or adenoma), it is a strong indication to remove the thyroid nodule. Good follow-up is a necessity.

Checking the serum levels of T4 after 1 month's therapy also ensures that the patient (e.g., one with multinodular goiter) has not become hyperthyroid because of autonomous or non-suppressible nodules. In such a patient with a non-suppressible nodule on L-thyroxine treatment the 24 hr I-131 uptake will be above 5% and the nodule(s) will be evident on scintiscan. It is wise to discontinue L-thyroxine in these patients since thyroid suppression will only lead to trouble.

THYROID CARCINOMA

Pathologically there are several forms of thyroid cancer but clinically thyroid carcinoma has four varieties: 1) papillary or mixed papillary-follicular carcinoma which represent 65-75% of all thyroid cancer; 2) follicular thyroid carcinoma (20-30%); 3) medullary thyroid carcinoma (5-10%); and 4) anaplastic carcinoma (rare, found in the elderly, responds poorly to any therapy, and is invariably fatal). Histology does bear on the prognosis. Papillary and mixed papillary-follicular carcinoma behave similarly and have a benign course; follicular carcinoma is more aggressive. The age of the patient at the time of diagnosis is a major prognostic feature. Young patients do well and seldom is there death from thyroid cancer below the age of 40. Papillary and mixed papillary-follicular cancers have a median age of onset at 35 whereas follicular occurs at a median age of 45 years (fig. 10.2).

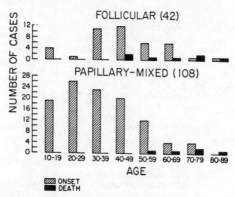

Figure 10.2 Age at onset of disease and death in 150 patients with well-differentiated thyroid carcinoma followed for > 15 yrs [Friedman EW, Schwartz AE: Well-differentiated thyroid cancer, in Krieger DT, Bardin CW (eds): Current Therapy in Endocrinology 1983-1984. Burlington, Ontario, BC Decker, 1983, p 93. with permission].

There is no difference in prognosis between men and women in this study (fig. 10.2), but others have reported males to have a slightly worse prognosis. The larger the size of the initial tumor the poorer the prognosis but regional node metastasis of papillary or mixed papillary-follicular carcinoma do not adversely affect prognosis.

Medullary thyroid carcinoma (MTC) of the parafollicular or C cells is a sporadic event in about 80% of cases, found at surgery for a solitary thyroid nodule. The average patient is 53 years old. The remainder of cases are familially inherited as an autosomal dominant trait. MTC is associated with pheochromocytoma (50% of cases) and hyperparathyroidism (10-25% of the patients) in multiple endocrine adenomatosis type IIa and with mucosal neuromatosis without hyperparathyroidism in multiple endocrine adenomatosis type IIb or III. The MTC associated with this latter syndrome (IIb) is very aggressive. Early detection of MTC in family members is possible and, with total thyroidectomy, represents the only way to cure this disease. <u>Calcitonin is the biochemical marker</u> of medullary thyroid carcinoma. Plasma calcitonin levels are drawn at 0 time and at 2, 3.5, 5, and 7 min after provocation with calcium gluconate iv (2 mg elemental Ca/kg over 1 min) followed by 10 sec bolus of pentagastrin 0.5 ug/kg. A rise of > 200 pg/ml is diagnostic of C-cell hyperplasia or MTC and surgery is essential to prevent overt disease.

<u>Management of Thyroid Carcinoma:</u> The management of thyroid carcinoma is controversial. The rarity, protracted course, and low mortality of well-differentiated carcinoma have made randomized treatment regimens difficult to perform. <u>It is generally agreed that the nodule should be removed and that thyroid suppressive therapy should be continued indefinitely.</u> How much thyroid to remove (one lobe vs total thyroidectomy) and the best method to provide follow-up are the unanswered variables.

Total thyroidectomy followed by 50-75 mCi of I-131 <u>one month</u> after surgery while the patient is hypothyroid (i.e., on no replacement thyroxine) will ablate any remaining functioning thyroid cells. Thyroid suppression with L-thyroxine is then instituted. <u>Six months</u> later after L-thyroxine is discontinued for at least one month a total body I-131 scan is performed as follows: the patient is given 1-2 mCi I-131 and then scintiscan 24 hrs and 48 hrs later. If the six month scan is negative, thyroxine suppression is reinstituted and the procedure repeated in <u>12-18 months.</u> If negative then, no more scans are performed <u>unless there</u> is evidence of local recurrence. If functioning tissue is identified on any scan then I-131 100-200 mCi is given, L-thyroxine reinstituted, and the body scan repeated six months later. This course is repeated as long as the scan is positive. Patients who are to receive > 30 mCi of I-131 are hospitalized in requirement of radiation safety standards. Patients are seen in yearly follow-up to assess the neck for recurrent nodules and to assure that levels of serum T4 are maintained with L-thyroxine. This combination of total thyroidectomy, I-131 ablation, and thyroid suppression offers effective therapy (fig. 10.3).

Functioning thyroid cells but not C cells make thyroglobulin which is found in the serum in small amounts. Once the thyroid is ablated (e.g., by total thyroidectomy or by large doses of I-131), no serum thyroglobulin is detectable. The presence of any measurable serum thyroglobulin after total ablation suggests recurrence of the disease since there should be no thyroid tissue remaining. The assay for serum thyroglobulin must be sensitive and specific to be useful.

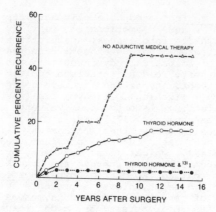

<u>Figure 10.3</u>   Cumulative recurrence rates for papillary and mixed papillary-follicular thyroid carcinoma according to type of medical therapy used postoperatively [Mazzaferri EL, Young RL, Oertel JE, Kemmerer WT, Page CP: Papillary thyroid carcinoma: the impact of therapy in 576 patients. <u>Medicine</u> 56:171, 1977. with permission].

The only reason for less surgery (i.e., sub-total thyroidectomy) at the initial operation is to avoid possible damage to the parathyroid glands which would render the patient chronically dependent on calcium and vitamin D (pages 123-124).   Up to 30% incidence of permanent hypoparathyroidism has been reported with total thyroidectomy.   This is not often a problem if the parathyroid glands are transplanted by an experienced surgeon.

The treatment of MTC is total thyroidectomy, ruling out pheochromocytoma (page 146) and hyperparathyroidism (page 117), and screening family members for the disease.

<u>HYPERTHYROIDISM</u>

Hyperthyroidism is the syndrome that develops after body tissues are exposed to increased concentrations of T4 and/or T3.   The clinical manifestations of hyperthyroidism can affect every organ.   The presentation varies with age, the classical symptoms and signs of hypermetabolism being seen in young and middle aged patients but less so in the elderly.   The degree of hyperthyroidism will also vary with the severity of the levels of T4 and T3.   The symptoms of hyperthyroidism can be related to <u>excessive sympathomimetic</u>

activity and to increased catabolic activity: nervousness
(irritability and emotional lability); increased
perspiration; heat intolerance; palpitations; weight loss;
dyspnea; fatigue and weakness; increased appetite;
hyperdefecation; menstrual dysfunction; and eye symptoms.
Signs of hyperthyroidism include goiter (thyroid enlargement), tremor, hyperkinesis, eye signs (exophthalmos,
lid retraction, lid lag), tachycardia (resting rate > 90;
atrial fibrillation), smooth and velvety skin, moist and
warm hands, onycholysis ("Plummer's nails"), and thyroid
bruit. In the elderly these classical signs are often
missing and one sees cardiac problems (heart failure and
tachydysrhythmias), weight loss, weakness, or anorexia. The
striking absence of the adrenergic and hyperkinetic symptoms
is sometimes called apathetic hyperthyroidism. When a
patient with hyperthyroidism presents with fever and
acceleration of these signs and symptoms the clinical
diagnosis of thyroid crisis is made (page 30). As with
thyroid diseases in general, hyperthyroidism is much more
common in females than males.

The diagnosis of hyperthyroidism is very easy when the
clinical disease is obvious. When the signs and symptoms
are minimal, the laboratory is helpful. The serum T4(RIA)
and T3U are usually elevated (pages 1-4) as is the serum
T3(RIA). The T3(RIA) is usually elevated to a greater
extent than the T4(RIA) and is sometimes the only abnormal
laboratory finding (i.e., T3-thyrotoxicosis). Hyperthyroidism has generalized effects on various tissues
producing numerous abnormal laboratory studies which revert
to normal when the hyperthyroidism resolves. Such findings
include hypercalcemia, abnormal liver function studies,
increase turnover and degradation of metabolites (e.g., an
increase in urinary 17-OHCS making one suspect Cushing's
syndrome). If subclinical hyperthyroidism is suspected, a
TRH study (page 5) should be performed.

The radionuclide thyroidal uptake or scan is not ordered
to make a diagnosis of hyperthyroidism but is helpful in
deciding the etiology of the hyperthyroidism.
Hyperthyroidism has many causes. These are listed in order
of decreasing frequency: 1) Graves' disease, 2)
thyroiditis, 3) toxic multinodular goiter, 4) toxic thyroid
adenoma, 5) exogenous hyperthyroidism (iatrogenic,
factitious, iodine-induced), 6) excess TSH (trophoblastic
tumors, pituitary tumor), and 7) ectopic thyroxine
production (struma ovarii and metastatic follicular thyroid
carcinoma).

GRAVES' DISEASE: Graves' disease is by far the most
common cause of hyperthyroidism with a female to male ratio
of 7 or 8 to 1. It is typically a disease of young women

(20-40 yrs) but may occur at any age. Graves' disease is distinguished clinically from other forms of hyperthyroidism by the presence of <u>diffuse thyroid enlargement,</u> <u>ophthalmopathy, and occasionally pretibial myxedema</u> although all these signs may be absent. Ophthalmopathy is present in 20-40% of patients with recent onset Graves' disease and may develop before hyperthyroidism ("euthyroid Graves' disease"), at the onset of hyperthyroidism (the usual case), or years later after the patient is euthyroid.

Graves' disease is an immunologic disorder of uncertain cause. Thyroid stimulating immunoglobulins (TSI) bind to the TSH receptors on follicular cells causing thyroidogenesis. When TSI levels decrease for any cause (most often spontaneous) the hyperthyroidism will go into remission. Genetic factors are important since 50% of monozygotic twins are concordant for hyperthyroidism and 5% of first-degree relatives have a history of hyperthyroidism. Currently the treatment of Graves' disease is directed at the thyroid gland rather than at the basic process which initiates the clinical disease.

<u>Treatment of Graves' disease:</u> The optimal therapy awaits a method that will treat the cause of this disorder. At present the best one can do is to control the hyperthyroidism with antithyroid drugs until the basic disease process undergoes spontaneous remission. Unfortunately spontaneous remission occurs in only 20-30% of patients in the United States. Therefore the clinician must decide on long-term anti-thyroid medication or on some form of ablative thyroid therapy such as radioactive iodine or, much less frequently, subtotal thyroidectomy.

<u>Antithyroid drugs:</u> The thionamides, propylthiouracil (PTU) and methimazole (Tapazole), block thyroid peroxidase and thus inhibit thyroid hormone biosynthesis. Both drugs have weak immunosuppressive effects and PTU has an inhibitory effect on the conversion of T4 to T3. The half-life of PTU is 1-2 hrs whereas methimazole is 6-8 hrs. Maximal effect is achieved with divided doses (q 6-8 hrs) especially with PTU but single doses may be effective in blocking thyroidogenesis. At present there are no reliable markers to define the population that will undergo spontaneous remission while on thionamide therapy. Clinically there are two groups that respond well to long term treatment--patients with a small thyroid gland and those whose hyperthyroidism is of very recent onset. These patients are treated with PTU 100-300 mg tid or methimazole 10-30 mg tid until the serum T3(RIA) is normal (usually 6-8 weeks after initiation) and then the dose is reduced or L-thyroxine is added to maintain euthyroid status. Patients are maintained on this therapy for 1-2 years before the drug

is discontinued although remissions have been reported when the drug is discontinued earlier. One of the most difficult aspects of therapy is to maintain patient compliance in taking medications. This is especially difficult with tid PTU which is only available as 50 mg tablets. Single or twice daily doses of methimazole 5-20 mg/day are a practical solution. Complications of thionamides are infrequent with rash being the most common problem (about 5% of the patients). Agranulocytosis is the most dreaded complication (0.2% of patients). Routine blood counts are not helpful or predictive of this toxic effect. The best policy is to tell the patient to come immediately for a complete blood count if there is fever, sore throat, or diarrhea. Other toxic reactions such as fever, myalgia, and lupus-like syndromes occur but remit as soon as the drug is discontinued.

Children and adolescents are usually managed with long-term thionamide therapy. Although the case is made that radioactive therapy is safe for children with hyperthyroidism, this is not universally accepted. Thionamides are used in treating the hyperthyroidism during pregnancy with lower doses than if the patient was not pregnant. These antithyroid medications cross the placenta and if given in large doses will inhibit the fetal thyroid gland. Doses of PTU up to 300 mg/day are generally safe. A mild degree of hyperthyroidism during pregnancy is usually well tolerated on thionamide treatment.

Short courses (1-3 months) of antithyroid drugs are used to reduce thyroid hormome levels and decrease the amount of hormone within the thyroid in preparation for ablative therapy.

<u>Radioactive iodine therapy:</u> I-131 therapy is the treatment of choice for most adults with Graves' disease. Patients who have failed long-term thionamide are also treated with I-131. It is safe, inexpensive, effective, and convenient; pregnancy is the only absolute contra-indication. Most patients are treated as outpatients. Elderly or especially ill patients are treated with thionamides until euthyroid then the thionamide discontinued for 4-7 days and I-131 given. This reduces the amount of thyroid hormone released after radiation injury and avoids the cardiovascular effects that may occur with a sudden surge in the serum levels of thyroid hormones. Younger patients may be treated while they are still hyperthyroid and covered with beta-adrenergic blockers (e.g., propranolol). The dose of I-131 is generally 5-15 mCi. The lower dose is associated with lower incidence of hypothyroidism but a higher incidence of unresolved hyperthyroidism. High doses of I-131 reverse these incidences. Within 6-12 weeks after I-131 the patient is generally euthyroid treatment and propranolol is

discontinued. If the patient is still hyperthyroid 6-12
months after I-131, a second treatment is necessary. The
incidence of hypothyroidism that develops depends on
treatment dose and ranges from 20% to 70%. Surveillance for
hypothyroidism must continue lifelong. Practically it is
easier to manage the patient if there is good ablation
leading to hypothyroidism. This complication is acceptable
since thyroid hormone replacement is easily managed with
L-thyroxine 0.1-0.2 mg/day at a cost of $.06 or less/day.
Good follow-up is necessary to treat hypothyroidism early or
to detect the recurrence of hyperthyroidism.

Surgery: Subtotal thyroidectomy is infrequently used in the
treatment of hyperthyroidism. Children who fail with
thionamides or patients who refuse radioactive medications
for personal reasons and the occasionally pregnant patient
with hyperthyroidism that cannot be managed with acceptable
doses of thionamides are treated with surgery. Before
operation, the patient is made euthyroid with thionamides
and potassium iodide drops. Pregnant patients are not given
the customary iodine preparation to reduce thyroid
vascularity since large fetal goiters may result.

Beta-adrenergic antagonists: The introduction of beta-
adrenergic antagonists has had a major influence of the
management of hyperthyroidism. Propranolol is the most
commonly used blocker. Propranolol alleviates but does not
totally resolve many of the symptoms of hyperthyroidism such
as tachycardia, sweating, tremor, heat intolerance, and
anxiety. The usual dose is 20-40 mg qid. As mentioned
above, propranolol is used as an adjunct to treatment with
I-131 until the therapeutic effect of I-131 is achieved. It
is also used in conjunction with potassium iodine and
thionamides in preparing patients with hyperthyroidism for
surgery. Propranolol is not prescibed if there is asthma.
Propranolol is especially useful in the treatment of thyroid
crisis (page 30).

Iodine: Inorganic iodine inhibits thyroid hormone synthesis
and release. Traditional doses of 5 to 10 drops of
saturated solution of potassium iodine tid in water or juice
will reduce the serum T4 and T3 by 50% within 7 to 14 days.
Then, T4 and T3 return to previous levels in most patients.
This escape phenomenon does not occur in a previously
damaged thyroid (e.g., radiation injury) and thus is useful
following I-131 therapy. Iodine is also used prior to
surgery for hyperthyroid subjects except in pregnancy.

THYROIDITIS: Two forms of thyroiditis may cause
hyperthyroidism: subacute (de Quervain's or granulomatous
or giant-cell) thyroiditis and painless thyroiditis.
Subacute thyroiditis is a painful condition which often

follows some respiratory illness. Thyroid follicules are disrupted and stored hormone is released causing hyperthyroid symptoms in 50% of the patients although levels of T4 are elevated in an even higher percentage. The radionuclide thyroidal uptake is characteristically very low (1-2% at 24 hrs) early in the course of this disorder. The hyperthyroidism is self-limited, lasting for only a few weeks. <u>Thionamides are not indicated and will not work.</u> Propranolol 20-40 mg qid is used for the hyperthyroid patient. Aspirin 650 mg qid is prescibed for treatment of the pain and is continued for several weeks after the pain resolves in an attempt to prevent recurrance of pain. If the pain is protracted, prednisone 20-40 mg/day is used for two-three weeks. <u>Painless thyroiditis</u> appears to be an increasing cause of hyperthyroidism. The gland is non-tender and only slightly enlarged. The radionuclide thyroidal may be low, normal, or increased. The etiology is uncertain. Treatment is the same as subacute thyroiditis except that salicylates are omitted.

<u>TOXIC MULTINODULAR GOITER:</u> Hyperthyroidism may develop as a late feature of multinodular goiter. Areas within the goiter become autonomous, i.e., not responsive to TSH. If sufficient tissue functions excessively, hyperthyroidism develops. The mechanism responsible for the autonomy is unknown. This is a disease of older patients (typically females over 60 yrs old). Large goiters may present with occasional retrosternal extension and tracheal compression. Many times the hyperthyroidism is mild and symptoms may be masked. Cardiac failure and atrial fibrillation may be present. The radionuclide scan shows patchy areas of increase activity. At times these patients become hyperthyroid after ingestion of organic iodine (often with T3-thyrotoxicosis). Others become toxic during thyroid suppressive therapy instituted in attempt to reduce the size of the goiter. In the latter two instances removing the offending agent is the first therapeutic move.

Toxic multinodular goiter is treated with ablative I-131 therapy. Patients are first given antithyroid medication to achieve euthyroidism. Thionamides are <u>not</u> prescribed for long-term therapy since spontaneous remissions rarely, if ever, occur. Large doses of I-131 (30-50 mCi) are necessary to ablate the thyroid and multiple doses are often necessary to control the hyperthyroidism. Surgery may be used especially for large goiters producing obstructive symptoms.

<u>TOXIC ADENOMA:</u> Toxic thyroid adenoma is a solitary benign lesion (follicular adenoma) that functions autonomously. The natural history is that of slow progressive growth except for an occasional hemorrhage into the adenoma leading to a decrease in the nodule size. Whether the patient

becomes hyperthyroid depends on the size of the nodule. The nodule usually has to be > 4 cm for hyperthyroidism to be evident. Smaller nodules may be hyperfunctioning on scan and produce enough thyroid hormone to suppress TSH and therefore reduce the uptake of radionuclide in surrounding normal thyroid tissue. T3-hyperthyroidism occurs in up to 50% of patients.

Treatment is with _surgery_ or _radioactive iodine._ For patients under 40 yrs old, surgery is recommended for those who have overt hyperthyroidism and prophylactically for those with large nodules. Hyperthyroid patients are prepared for surgery either with antithyroid drugs or with the combination of propranolol and inorganic iodine. Most older patients will receive I-131 therapy. Large doses of I-131 (20-25 mCi) are necessary to ablate the adenoma. Hypothyroidism is rare following I-131 therapy for toxic thyroid adenoma and toxic multinodular goiter whereas it is the rule after treatment for Graves' disease. Smaller autonomous nodules in euthyroid patients need not be treated, but the patients must be followed carefully and thyroid function measured at yearly intervals.

Exogenous Hyperthyroidism:

Iatrogenic hyperthyroidism will developed in patients receiving larger than replacement doses of thyroid hormones. This is common with doses of L-thyroxine in excess of 0.3 mg and is even more common when T3 or a combination T4 and T3 is used. Assessment of the thyroid status by measuring serum T4(RIA) may be misleading in patients treated with T3 or combined T3-T4 preparations. Occasional patients with multinodular goiter on seemingly appropiate suppressive doses of L-thyroxine (e.g., 0.15 mg/day) will have high T4(RIA) levels. This is the time to determine whether there is autonomous function within the adenomatous nodules (contributing to the hyperthyroxinemia) or whether the dose of L-thyroxine itself is too much. A radionuclide uptake and scan should be performed. If the uptake is > 5% or if functioning nodule(s) are found, L-thyroxine is discontinued. If the uptake is < 5% and no hyperfunctioning areas are indentified, then the dose of L-thyroxine is reduced.

Factitious hyperthyroidism: Some patients with personality disorders (often paramedical personel) may induce hyperthyroidism by the intentional self-administration of thyroid hormones. In these cases, the thyroid gland is not enlarged nor are there any signs of ophthalmopathy or pretibial myxedema. The serum T4(RIA) or T3(RIA) or both are elevated depending on which thyroid hormone preparation is ingested. The TSH response to TRH is

blunted and the radionuclide thyroidal uptake is low.
Psychiatric referral may be necessary for these patients.

Iodine-induced hyperthyroidism: In areas of endemic
goiter due to iodine deficiency, dietary iodine
supplementation will decrease the size of the thyroid.
Nevertheless, this treatment induces hyperthyroidism in a
subset of patients who have a preexisting thyroid
abnormality. Iodine-induced hyperthyroidism also occurs in
nonendemic regions in patients who have multinodular goiter
or thyroid adenoma. These patients become hyperthyroid
several weeks after ingestion of large doses of inorganic
iodine (e.g., amiodarone) or radiographic contrast agents.
Because the pool of iodine is expanded, the radionuclide
thyroidal uptake may be low. Symptomatic treatment with
propranolol and withdrawal of any iodine-containing
medication is indicated.

TSH producing tumors are a very rare cause of
hyperthyroidism. Several cases of a pituitary tumor
producing TSH have been reported. Trophoblastic tumors such
as choriocarcinoma, hydatidiform moles, or embryonal
carcinoma of the testes produce high levels of chorionic
gonadotropin which weakly cross reacts with the TSH receptor
of the thyroid follicular cell. In these cases, overt
hyperthyroidism is rare.

HYPOTHYROIDISM

Hypothyroidism develops when there is inadequate effect
of thyroid hormone on body tissues. Greater than 99.9% of
the time hypothyroidism is caused by deficient production of
thyroid hormones by the thyroid gland leading to low serum
levels of T4. Very very rarely hypothyroidism is due to
failure of tissues to respond to normal or raised levels of
thyroid hormones (e.i., peripheral resistance). In
hypothyroidism the tissues are infiltrated by hydrophilic
mucopolysaccharides. This leads to the non-pitting edema
(most marked in the skin of the eyelids and hands) termed
myxedema.

The clinical spectrum of hypothyroidism ranges from
subtle and subclinical disease to gross and obvious changes
which have developed over years. Classical symptoms of
hypothyroidism are: marked cold intolerance (prefers warm
room, extra clothes, sleeps with blanket during the warm
months); weakness (incresed tiredness, slowing down); muscle
cramps, aching, and stiffness; hoarseness, decreased
hearing, and paresthesias (a result of myxedematous changes
in the vocal cords, middle ear and eighth cranial nerve, and
carpal tunnel syndrome respectively); mild weight gain

despite normal appetite; constipation and ileus; dry skin and decreased perspiration; and somnolence. Frequent <u>signs</u> include skin which is rough, scaly, dry, cool to the touch, and pallid or yellow tinted (the result of anemia or hypercarotenemia due to impaired conversion of carotene to vitamin A); non-pitting edema of the eyelids, hands, and feet; slow movements and slowness of thought (a dementia which responses to T4 replacement); <u>slow relaxation time of deep tendon reflexes;</u> and cardiovascular signs (bradycardia, cardiac failure, pericardial effusion, and <u>hypertension).</u> Severe hypothyroidism can lead to coma and respiratory compromise (see myxedema coma, page 28). Congenital hypothyroidism is associated with mental retardation and characteristic facies. Juvenile hypothyroidism is characterized by epiphyseal dysgenesis and short stature. Goiter may or may not be present depending on the etiology of the hypothyroidism.

Hypothyroidism has many causes but most involve thyroidal (primary) hypofunction either with insufficient amount of functional tissue (e.g., primary atrophy, chronic thyroiditis, prior I-131 treatment or surgery, thyroid agenesis) or some form of defective biosynthesis of thyroid hormone (e.g., iodine deficiency, congenital defects of trapping or organification of iodine, excessive antithyroid medications, or iodine excess). Secondary hypothyroidism related to pituitary disease (e.g., pituitary tumor) is usually but not always obvious since other signs of hypopituitarism are often present. If the serum T4(RIA) and T3U are low and the TSH is low as well, one should examine the hypothalmic-pituitary axis. Clinically primary hypothyroidism can be classified by whether a <u>goiter is or is not present and by whether the hypothyroidism follows some ablative procedure.</u>

Hypothyroidism is confirmed by finding a low serum T4(RIA) and T3U. In all forms of primary hypothyroidism the serum TSH is elevated and should always be measured since a low value implies pituitary disease (pages 66-67). Antibodies to thyroid microsomes and thyroglobulin are usually present in autoimmune thyroid disease (primary atrophy and Hashimoto's thyroiditis). Anemia of some form (microcytic, from menstrual loss in premenopausal females; normochromic normocytic, from decreased erythropoietin production; macrocytic, from associated pernicious anemia) is often present. The enzymes creatine kinase and aspartate aminotransferase are released from muscle and may be markedly elevated in the serum. Serum cholesterol and triglycerides are often raised. The sella turcica may be enlarged in long-term hypothyroidism. The ECG may demonstrate low voltage if pericardial effusion is present. <u>Serum T3(RIA) levels are not helpful since over half of the</u>

patients with hypothyroidism have levels within the normal range.

Non-goitrous hypothyroidism:

Spontaneous primary thyroid atrophy is a common cause of hypothyroidism. No goiter is present. It is found more often in females than males (6:1) and increases in frequency with age. There is loss of thyroid tissue as a result of autoimmune destruction leading to fibrosis and atrophy of the thyroid. Primary atrophy represents one end of the spectrum of autoimmune thyroid disease; at the other is chronic autoimmune (Hashimoto's) thyroiditis in which there is marked proliferation of lymphocytes and acinar formation leading to goiter. In most cases thyroid failure has been present for months or years prior to diagnosis. There may be associated failure of other endocrine organs including pernicious anemia, diabetes mellitus, hypogonadism, hypoparathyroidism, and Addison's disease.

Goitrous hypothyroidism:

Chronic autoimmune thyroiditis (Hashimoto's thyroiditis) is characterized by a diffuse enlargement of the thyroid gland and high titers of thyroid autoantibodies. This condition is the most common cause of goitrous hypothyroidism in iodine-replete parts of the world. The titers of autoantibodies are much higher than in primary thyroid atrophy. Histologically the thyroid has large amounts of lymphocyte infiltration with areas of marked follicular hypertrophy and/or numerous oxyphilic cells (Hurthle cells). Failure of other endocrine organs may be associated with Hashimoto's thyroiditis. For example, the combination of chronic lymphocytic thyroiditis and idiopathic adrenal insufficiency is known as Schmidt's syndrome.

Drug-induced hypothyroidism may be secondary to lithium carbonate, iodine, or antithyroid drugs. Lithium inhibits the release of thyroid hormone and is one of the common causes of goiter but rarely causes hypothyroidism. Iodine may cause goiter in susceptible subjects (i.e., those with some underlying thyroid abnormality) and lead to hypothyroidism. Typically this is seen in patients with chronic respiratory disease taking expectorants containing potassium iodide.

Hypothyroidism due to iodine deficiency is a common problem in areas of endemic goiter in certain parts of the world. It is almost never seen in the United States.

Dyshormonogenesis: Inherited disorders of dyshormonogenesis are rare and are typically inherited as an autosomal recessive trait. The most common defect is associated with progressive hearing loss leading to deafness and goiter due to an inability to organify iodine (Pendred's syndrome).

Post-ablative hypothyroidism may follow surgery or radioactive iodine therapy and represents a frequent cause of hypothyroidism. In fact, post I-131 induced hypothyroidism is the most common cause of hypothyroidism in the author's clinic.

Treatment of hypothyroidism

Therapy for primary hypothyroidism is simple. L-thyroxine is routinely prescibed in a dose of 2 ug/kg body weight/day with the average replacement dose being approximately 150-200 ug/day. The half-life of T4 is 6 to 8 days which allows for stable and constant serum levels of T4. The advantages of synthetic L-thyroxine include the following: assured potency; single daily dose; inexpensive ($0.06 or less/day); constant levels of serum T4; and the ability to assess adequacy of replacement by measuring serum T4(RIA). Absorption of L-thyroxine is somewhat variable from individual to individual. Most patients will normalize their TSH with 0.15 mg of L-thyroxine/day and nearly all with 0.2 mg/day. Since 80% of body T3 is derived by conversion of T4, serum T3(RIA) levels are normal in the patient taking replacement L-thyroxine.

The regimen for each patient must be individualized. For the young, mildly hypothyroid patient one may start with full replacement dose (e.g., L-thyroxine 0.15 mg/day) remembering that it will take nearly a month for the full effects of T4 to be realized. For the severely hypothyroid patient, gradual replacement is indicated in order to avoid cardiovascular problems. L-thyroxine 0.025 mg/day is prescribed for two-three weeks and then increased by 0.025 mg/day every two-three weeks until maintenance dose is reached.

T3 is not routinely used for several reasons: peaks of T3 following gut absorption are much higher than normal serum T3(RIA); T3 must be taken tid; T3 is considerable more expensive than L-thyroxine; and serum T4(RIA) cannot be used to assess replacement therapy.

A problem with all medications that must be taken chronically is patient compliance. Education as to the importance of renewing prescriptions and annual follow-up to assess long-term therapy can not be overemphasized. Elderly hypothyroid patients may forget to take their medications so it is important that someone be responsible for avoiding this problem.

Withdrawal of thyroid medication

There are large numbers of patients who have been prescibed thyroid medication for vague symptoms (e.g., weakness, fatigue, menstrual dysfunction) without any laboratory documentation of hypothyroidism. The best way to find out whether the patient needs to continue thyroid meds is to discontinue the preparation. Six weeks later serum T4(RIA), T3U, and TSH are measured. If the patient is symptomatic _and_ the lab values confirm hypothyroidism, then reinstitute thyroid using L-thyroxine as discussed above. If the patient has no symptoms and the TSH is slightly elevated, wait several more weeks until symptoms develop and TSH remains elevated prior to starting L-thyroxine. If the lab values are normal after six weeks off thyroid preparation, no further thyroid medication is prescribed. Follow-up 3-6 months later should confirm that no replacement is necessary.

Simple non-toxic goiter

Simple goiter is found often in young women who present with enlargement of the anterior neck. The thyroid may be just palpable or moderately enlarged. The gland is usually soft, non-tender, and diffusely enlarged. No nodules are palpable. The patient is asymptomatic and is chemically euthyroid. Thyroid autoantibodies are absent or present in low titer. The etiology is rarely discernible. The patient may be merely followed to see if the thyroid will continue to enlarge or may be begun on thyroid suppression if the gland is already modestly enlarged. Thyroid suppression will usually decrease the size of the thyroid and therapy is continued indefinitely. Inform the patient that discontinuation of thyroid meds may be followed by recurrence of the goiter.

Euthyroid sick

Thyroid tests are often ordered to screen for thyroid disease in patients who have weakness, anxiety, tachycardia, and weight loss. The majority of these patients do not have primary thyroid disease. Euthyroid sick is a term designated for those patients with nonthyroidal illnesses who have abnormal thyroid tests and can be classified into the following categories: 1) low T3 syndrome; 2) low T3 and low T4 syndrome; 3) high T4 syndrome; and 4) a mixed form in which a combination of abnormalites may be found.

Low T3 syndrome is the most common of the euthyroid sick abnormalities but is usually not identified since most screening studies do not measure T3(RIA). The serum T3(RIA)

is low and the serum T4(RIA) is normal. The patient is
clinically euthyroid.   The serum T3(RIA) may be low in many
circumstances: <u>systemic illnesses</u> (e.g., liver disease,
acute   febrile   illnesses,   renal   failure,   neoplastic
disorders, burns, and congestive heart failure); <u>starvation;
major surgery; and following the administration of some
drugs</u> (dexamethasone, cholecystographic dyes, amiodarone,
high doses of propranolol, and thionamides). The common
factor in all these conditions is <u>reduced extrathyroidal
conversion of T4 to T3.</u> The conversion of reverse T3 (rT3)
to T2 is impaired leading to increased levels of serum rT3.
The TSH is normal and the free T4 measured by dialysis
techniques is normal or high. The low T3 resolves when the
underlying illness clears.

The <u>low T3 and low T4 syndrome</u> is usually identified
because a low serum T4(RIA) found on screening for thyroid
disease.   The free thyroid index (FTI) is often low as well.
These patients are severely ill and the clinical assessment
to totally exclude hypothyroidism is difficult. However,
careful history and physical examination will <u>not</u> reveal the
typical features of hypothyroidism (page 108).   Free T4
levels are normal or high. Serum TSH and TRH testing (i.e.,
TSH response to TRH) are normal. Patients who have a low T3
and low T4 generally do not do well when the T4(RIA) is < 3
ug/dl (mortality approaches 84%) and underscores the
severity of the nonthyroidal illness found in this set of
patients.   There no evidence that treatment with L-thyroxine
will help these patients. In fact, most experts believe the
low T4 and low T3 levels are an adaptive mechanism in order
to spare protein catabolism under these circumstances.

The major cause of elevated T4 <u>(high T4 syndrome)</u> in
euthyroid sick patients is increased concentrations of TBG
produced in certain liver diseases (e.g., acute viral
hepatitis, chronic active hepatitis, and primary biliary
cirrhosis) and acute intermittent porphyria. The TRH study
is normal in these patients. Hyperthyroxinemia can be found
in patients who have recently ingested radiographic contrast
agents [ipodate (Oragrafin) or iopanoic acid (Telepaque)].
These agents compete with 5'deiodinase and impair T4 to T3
conversion which leads to elevated serum T4(RIA) levels.
The T4 returns to normal within 6-8 weeks. High doses of
propranolol occasionally cause an elevated T4 presumably by
inhibiting the conversion of T4 to T3. Another cause of
hyperthyroxinemia which there is no evidence of clinical
hyperthyroidism is familial dysalbumenic hyperthyroxinemia,
a disorder in which albumin binds T4 abnormally leading to
raised levels of T4(RIA) and normal T3U. Again the TRH
study is normal in each of these conditions of elevated T4.

References

Berger CL, Well SA Jr, Mendelsohn G, Baylin SB: Medullary thyroid carcinoma, in Krieger DT, Bardin CW (eds): Current Therapy in Endocrinology 1983-1984. Burlington, Ontario, BC Decker, 1983, pp 98-104.

Burch W: A method of fine-needle aspiration thyroid biopsy. Ann Intern Med 98:1023, 1983.

Burch WM: A method of aspirating thyroid cysts. Surg Gynecol Obstet 148: 95, 1979.

Burrow GN: The thyroid: nodules and neoplasia, in Felig P, Baxter JD, Broadus AE, Frohman LA (eds): Endocrinology and Metabolism. New York, McGraw-Hill, 1981, pp 351-382.

Chopra IJ: Thyroid function in nonthyroidal illnesses. Ann Intern Med 98:946, 1983.

Fradkin JE, Wolff J: Iodide-induced thyrotoxicosis. Medicine 62:1, 1983.

Friedman EW, Schwartz AE: Well-differentiated thyroid cancer, in Krieger DT, Bardin CW (eds): Current Therapy in Endocrinology 1983-1984. Burlington, Ontario, BC Decker, 1983, pp 92-98.

Mazzaferri EL, Young RL, Oertel JE, Kemmerer WT, Page CP: Papillary thyroid carcinoma: the impact of therapy in 576 patients. Medicine 56:171, 1977.

Ruiz M, Rajatanavin R, Young RA et al: Familial dysalbuminemic hyperthyroxinemia: a syndrome that can be confused with thyrotoxicosis. N Engl J Med 306:635, 1982.

Schimmel M, Utiger RD: Thyroidal and peripheral production of thyroid hormones: review of recent findings and their clinical implications. Ann Intern Med 87:760, 1977.

Spaulding SW, Utiger RD: The thyroid: physiology, hyperthyroidism, hypothyroidism, and the painful thyroid, in Felig P, Baxter JD, Broadus AE, Frohman LA (eds): Endocrinology and Metabolism. New York, McGraw-Hill, 1981, pp 281-350.

Van Herle AJ, Rich P, Ljung BME, Ashcraft MW, Solomon DH: The thyroid nodule. Ann Intern Med 96:221, 1982.

Chapter 11

Calcium Disorders

HYPERCALCEMIA

Normal serum calcium ranges from 8.5 mg/dl to 10.5 mg/dl in most laboratories. Care should be taken to interpret serum calcium in view of the protein concentration as discussed on pages 20 and 31. Elevated serum calciums are frequently found even in asymptomatic subjects. Over 50% of patients with hypercalcemia are identified by the serendipitous finding of an elevated serum calcium on biochemical sceening profile studies. Others present with symptoms and signs that can be directly attributed to an underlying disease (e.g., bone pain related to osseous metastasis or renal stones due to hyperparathyroidism).

Symptoms of hypercalcemia are related to the degree and duration of the hypercalcemia. Patients with serum calciums < 11.0 mg/dl are rarely symptomatic in regards to calcium itself although they may be very symptomatic related to any underlying disease (e.g., malignancy). Levels of serum calcium between 11.0 and 14.0 mg/dl may or may not be associated with symptoms. Hypercalcemia above 14.0 mg/dl is invariably associated with symptoms and the risk of developing severe organ damage is significant at these levels. Symptoms of hypercalcemia are not specific. General symptoms of weakness, fatigue, impaired mental concentration are frequent. Polyuria is an early manifestation; hypercalcemia impairs the ability of the renal tubules to respond to vasopressin (ADH) so that urine cannot be maximally concentrated. Neurologic symptoms of poor recent memory, depression, muscle weakness, and lethargy can progress to stupor and coma (page 31). Gastrointestinal complaints include anorexia, nausea, vomiting, and constipation.

Signs for hypercalcemia are uncommon or non-specific. Band keratopathy, a manifestation of metastatic calcification, is probably the most specific sign of chronic hypercalcemia. Band keratopathy occurs in the medial and lateral margins of the cornea adjacent to the scleral limbus whereas the deposition of arcus senilis begins superiorly and inferiorly and extends around the margins of the cornea giving the arcus circularis (annulus senilis). Arcus circularis is separated from the limbus by a clear space within the cornea. This space is often obliterated and filled with whitish deposits in band keratopathy. The predominant cardiovascular sign of hypercalcemia is hypertension. Shortened QT interval on the ECG and increased sensitivity to digitalis is also seen. Renal signs relate to the inability to concentrate urine, renal stones, and renal insufficiency. Pancreatitis and peptic ulcer disease are associated with hypercalcemia as are gout and pseudogout. Dehydration leading to hypercalcemic crisis (page 31) may be the only sign of severe hypercalcemia.

Hypercalcemia has multiple etiologies. Greater than 90% of patients have either primary hyperparathyroidism or malignancy as the cause of hypercalcemia. Other causes are listed in the following table.

Table 11.1   Causes of Hypercalcemia

Primary hyperparathyroidism
    Sporadic (90-95% of the cases of hyperparathyroidism)
    Familial syndromes (MEN I and MEN IIa)
        MEN I-(tumors of pituitary, pancreas, parathyroid)
        MEN IIa-(medullary thyroid carcinoma, hyperparathy-
            roidism, pheochromocytoma)
Neoplastic diseases
    Local osteolysis (breast and lung carcinoma metastatic
                 to bone and myeloma)
    Humoral hypercalcemia of malignancy

Endocrine disorders
    Hyperthyroidism
    Adrenal Insufficiency
    Familial hypocalciuric hypercalcemia

Medications
    Thiazide diuretics
    Vitamin D and rarely vitamin A intoxication
    Milk-alkali syndrome
    Lithium

Granulomatous diseases
    Sarcoidosis
    Beryllosis, tuberculosis, coccidioidomycosis

Miscellaneous
    Immobilization (associated with high bone turnover
            rates such as in children or Paget's disease)
    Recovery phase of acute renal failure (rare)
    Idiopathic hypercalcemia of infancy (rare)

HYPERPARATHYROIDISM: The   prevalence of hyperparathyroidism
is about 1 in 1000.   This disease affects females more often
than   males   in a ratio of about 2-3 to 1.   Most patients are
over   50   yrs old.   Hyperparathyroidism is caused by a parathyroid   adenoma in about 85% of the cases, by hyperplasia of
the   parathyroid   glands   (15%),   or   rarely   by parathyroid
carcinoma.   The   natural   history   of hyperparathyroidism is
uncertain   since   patients with minimal or biochemical (serum
calcium < 1 mg/dl above   normal) disease are treated with
parathyroidectomy and cured.   Prior to the introduction of
screening   serum   profiles,   clinical   clues   to
hyperparathyroidism   related   to renal stones (64% of cases),
bone   disease   such as osteitis fibrosa cystica (page 133) in
about   20% of   the   cases,   peptic ulcer disease (12% of the
cases),   or   hypertension   (6%).   Asymptomatic patients
comprised about 7% of these cases.   These complications of
parathyroid   hormone   excess are still seen but the frequency
of each has changed because patients are identified earlier
before   such   manifestations   are   evident.   It is known that
primary hyperparathyroidism   is   a   chronic disease and that
patients   can   have   asymptomatic hypercalcemia over long
periods of time (years).

The   diagnosis   of   hyperparathyroidism   depends   on
demonstrating persistent hypercalcemia in the absence of
other   causes   of   hypercalcemia.   A history of hypercalcemia
for   over   a   year   in   the   absence of weight loss and other
systemic   symptoms   excludes   the   other   major   cause   of
hypercalcemia-- neoplastic disease.   Phosphate excretion and
nephrogenous   cyclic AMP are increased (page 21), but these
studies   are   rarely   necessary   if a careful evaluation has
excluded   other   causes of hypercalcemia. Medical records of
previous   lab studies are well worth the trouble of obtaining
to   see   if   prior   hypercalcemia   can   be   documented.
Measurement   of   serum   parathyroid   hormone   (RIA) may be
helpful   in   questionable   cases.   PTH (RIA) should not be
considered   with   the   same respect or validity as an RIA for
growth   hormone in acromegaly or insulin in the evaluation of
hypoglycemia   (page 21).   Other biochemical studies that are
helpful   but   not diagnostic include hypophosphatemia (< 3.0
mg/dl),   serum   chloride   > 106 meq/l, serum phosphorus/serum
chloride   ratio > 33, elevated serum alkaline phosphatase, or
a   calcium-phosphate   renal stone.   Radiographic findings are
rare   in   the   asymptomatic   patient   but   subperiosteal
resorption   of   the   phalanges   and   metacarpals is virtually
pathognomonic of hyperparathyroidism (page 133).

The   only   effective   therapy   for   hyperparathyroidism is
surgical   removal   of   the parathyroid adenoma/hyperplasia.
The   presence   of   severe hypercalcemia, renal disease, renal
stones,   bone   pain,   peptic ulcer, and hypertension are
indications   for   neck   exploration.   Likewise, patients with

MEN I and IIa who have hypercalcemia should have parathyroidectomy. Although the natural history for asymptomatic patients with lesser degrees of hypercalcemia (< 12 mg/dl) is unknown, at least 25% of these patients will developed some complication attributable to hyperparathyroidism (e.g., decreased creatinine clearance, renal stone, nephrocalcinosis, hypertension, etc.) within five years of followup. Unfortunately there is no marker to define which patients will develop complications related to hypercalcemia. <u>The critical factor in the management of the hyperparathyroidism is the availability of an experienced parathyroid surgeon.</u> In most centers such a surgeon is available and thus neck exploration is routinely advised even in asymptomatic patients. The surgery is delicate but relatively benign. Most patients are discharged cured on the 2nd or 3rd post operative day. Age itself is not a contraindication to surgery. Hypocalcemia is the major problem following surgery in the patient who has <u>bone disease and elevated serum alkaline phosphatase preoperatively.</u> Such patients will generally need large doses of calcium iv (page 34), oral calcium, and possibly short-acting calcitriol (0.5-1.0 ug bid) for several weeks postoperatively until the "hungry bones" have reached a state of equilibrium after escaping the resorptive effects of chronic hyperparathyroidism. By then the serum alkaline phosphatase and serum phosphorus will have returned to normal and calcium supplementation can be discontinued. A few patients will have permanent hypoparathyroidism and need indefinite treatment (page 123). Recurrence of hyperparathyroidism is most likely in the patients with parathyroid hyperplasia (often the familial syndromes associated with hypercalcemia).

<u>There is no satisfactory medical therapy for primary hyperparathyroidism.</u> However medical therapy is used in two well-defined areas. <u>Life-threatening hypercalcemia</u> is managed medically with hydration and agents that will acutely lower the serum calcium (pages 31-32). Patients who are <u>unacceptable surgical risks</u> are medically treated. Many of these patients have no symptoms directly related to hypercalcemia <u>as long as adequate hydration is assured.</u> Any illness such as viral gastroenteritis can lead to dehydration and hypercalcemic crisis and the patient must be warned to get medical attention. <u>Oral phosphates</u> given initially in small doses to avoid diarrhea and increased to 1-2 gm qid are reasonable agents to use in an attempt to lower the serum calcium. Careful monitoring of renal function, serum potassium, and serum phosphorus (maintained below 5 mg/dl to minimize ectopic calcification) are necessary. <u>Estrogen</u> (Premarin 0.625-1.25 mg/day) may be used since estrogen is known to inhibit PTH-induced bone resorption. Despite these measures there is no ideal

therapy for these hypercalcemic patients who often have underlying illnesses such as hypertension or congestive heart failure which complicate therapy with salt loading and digitalis.

NEOPLASTIC DISEASES: Hypercalcemia of malignancy may be caused by direct osteolysis due to bony metastases (breast and lung carcinoma most common) or to myeloma which makes a factor that stimulates osteoclasts to resorb bone (osteoclast activating factor or OAF). In many patients with malignancy the hypercalcemia cannot be attributed to tumor invasion of the bone. These patients have humoral hypercalcemia of malignancy (HHM). The factor(s) responsible for the hypercalcemia are unknown. Ectopic production of PTH by tumor appears unlikely since most investigators have not demonstrated any PTH elevation associated with this syndrome. Furthermore, tumors known to be associated with HHM do not make any mRNA that hybridizes with native PTH mRNA suggesting that ectopic PTH production is not the cause of HHM. Prostaglandin E may be one of the factors but prostaglandin synthesis inhibitors such as indomethacin are not very successful in treating HHM.

ENDOCRINE-RELATED HYPERCALCEMIA: Thyrotoxicosis is associated with increased bone resorption and increased bone turnover. The hypercalcemia is modest and abates as the hyperthyroidism resolves with treatment. Acute adrenal insufficiency is rarely associated with hypercalcemia which resolves with glucocorticoid treatment. The mechanism for the hypercalcemia of Addison's disease is not understood. Pheochromocytoma may be associated with hypercalcemia as part of the MEN syndromes. The pheochromocytoma is managed surgically before parathyroid exploration. Familial hypocalciuric hypercalcemia is distinct from primary hyperparathyroidism in several respects: age, urine calcium, complications, and response to surgery. This is a familial disorder in which most patients will be < 20 yrs of age. Urine calcium excretion is inappropiately low for the degree of hypercalcemia, often less than 100 mg/day (most hyperparathyroid patients excrete > 250 mg/day). Complications of hypercalcemia such as nephrolithiasis and peptic ulcer disease are rare. Furthermore, subtotal parathyroidectomy does not cure the hypercalcemia although total parathyroidectomy does lead to hypocalcemia. The pathophysiology of this unusual disorder is not known. The management of this autosomal dominant syndrome is first "do no harm." Since complications are rare and surgery does not correct the hypercalcemia, operation is avoided. Identification of family members with this disorder and patient education are where efforts need to be directed.

MEDICATION-RELATED HYPERCALCEMIA: Thiazide diuretics and related drugs (e.g., chlorthalidone) are natriuretic but not calciuretic leading to decreased calcium excretion in most patients.   The hypercalcemic effect of thiazides also occurs in anephric patients indicating other organs are affected by diuretics as well. The hypercalcemia (usually < 11.5 mg/dl) should resolve within two-three weeks after discontinuation of the medication. If hypercalcemia persists, then primary hyperparathyroidism is the most likely diagnosis. Vitamin D intoxication may be found in health faddists or as a complication of therapy for hypoparathyroidism, renal osteodystrophy, hypophosphatemic rickets, or intestinal malabsorption.   It is particularly likely with ergo-calciferol, vitamin D2, which is stored in fat depots for months.   Treatment consists of discontinuation of vitamin D and calcium supplements, hydration and diuresis (furosemide), and hydrocortisone (100 to 200 mg/day) or equivalent steroid until the patient is normocalcemic. Vitamin A intoxication may occur with doses > 50,000 U/day. Pharmacologic doses of vitamin A causes osteoclastic bone resorption.   Any patient with a skin disorder may be receiving vitamin A, so history is important. The treatment is as for vitamin D intoxication. Milk-alkali syndrome results from ingestion of large amounts of calcium carbonate and calcium bicarbonate usually in the treatment of peptic ulcer disease. This syndrome is unusual today because of the use of non-absorbable antacids. Renal insufficiency, hypocalciuria, alkalosis, and hyperphosphatemia are invariably present. The pathogenesis of lithium-induced hypercalcemia is obscure.

GRANULOMATOUS DISEASE: Sarcoidosis is by far the most common cause of hypercalcemia within this group. About 10% of patients with active sarcoidosis have hypercalcemia but over 40% have hypercalciuria, often with nephrolithiasis. Patients with sarcoidosis are known to have an increased conversion of 25-hydroxyvitamin D to 1,25-dihydroxyvitamin D.   This correlates with the observation that sarcoid patients become hypercalcemic on small doses of vitamin D2 (10,000 U/day) whereas most normal subjects tolerate 10 times this amount without overt hypercalcemia. Hyper-calcemia is more prevalent in sarcoidosis during the summer months when endogenous production of vitamin D is increased. Serum levels of 1,25-dihydroxyvitamin D are elevated in active sarcoidosis, but the mechanism responsible for this conversion is not yet understood.   Treatment with glucocorticoids should be correlated with the activity of the underlying granulomatous disease.

IMMOBILIZATION: Immobilization of patients with Paget's disease (page 134) or other states of high bone turnover (as in children) is also likely to result in hypercalcemia as well as hypercalciuria. Treatment consists of hydration and early ambulation.

HYPOCALCEMIA

A low serum ionized calcium produces characteristic symptoms. Since about half of the total serum calcium is bound to protein, a low serum calcium should be anticipated in cases of low albumin. Acute hyperventilation leads to alkalosis which lowers the ionized calcium without changing the total serum calcium. The severity and duration of the hypocalcemia will dictate the clinical presentation. Acute hypocalcemia is much more likely to be symptomatic than chronic hypocalcemia despite equivalent levels of serum calcium. Signs and symptoms of neuromuscular irritability predominate and include weakness, muscle cramps, paresthesias of the hands and feet, and tetany. Epileptiform seizures and laryngospasm are common presentations in children. Signs of latent tetany include Chvostek's sign (tapping facial nerve over the parotid elicits a twitch at the angle of the mouth) and Trousseau's sign (inflating the sphygmomanometer about 20 mm Hg above the systolic blood pressure for 3 minutes produces carpal spasm--flexion of the wrist and metacarpophalangeal joints and adduction of the thumb). A faint Chvostek's sign is present in about 10% of the normal population but development of a strong Chvostek's sign after neck surgery suggests hypocalcemia. Trousseau's sign is a more reliable indicator of hypocalcemia. Tetany is not specific for hypocalcemia and may be seen in hypomagnesemia, in hypokalemia, and in respiratory alkalosis as mentioned above. Serum phosphate is usually high in hypoparathyroidism. Calcification of the basal ganglia is seen in about half of the children with chronic hypocalcemia and may be associated with extrapyramidal signs of parkinsonism and choreoathetosis. Cataracts are commom in chronic hypocalcemia; the cause is unknown but treatment of the hypocalcemia will stop their progression. Idiopathic hypoparathyroidism may be associated with mucocutaneous candidiasis.

The differential diagnosis of hypocalcemia includes: hypoparathyroidism due to PTH deficiency or resistance (pseudohypoparathyroidism); hypomagnesemia; pancreatitis; acute phosphate intoxication; and vitamin D deficiency, malabsorption, and renal insufficiency as discussed in chapter 12 on metabolic bone disease.

HYPOPARATHYROIDISM: Deficiency of PTH may be complication of neck surgery (thyroid, parathyroid, surgery for carcinoma of larynx). Surgical hypoparathyroidism is the most common cause of hypoparathyroidism. Hypocalcemia after surgery for hyperparathyroidism is usually related to the "hungry bone syndrome." These patients will have hypophosphatemia as opposed to the typical hyperphosphatemia of true parathyroid deficiency. The management of surgical hypoparathyroidism is generally much easier than idiopathic hypoparathyroidism since smaller doses of vitamin D or even calcium supplements alone will correct the hypocalcemia, presumably some PTH is still being produced. Idiopathic hypoparathyroidism is rare and may occur alone or be associated with autoimmune polyglandular failure. Most cases are sporadic and occur before the age of 15 yrs. Hypoparathyroidism is the result of total atrophy of the parathyroid glands. The associated features of autoimmune disease include hypoparathyroidism, Addison's disease, and moniliasis (HAM syndrome) as well hypothyroidism, pernicious anemia, ovarian failure, vitiligo, and myasthenia gravis. The diagnosis of hypoparathyroidism is confirmed by demonstrating a rise in serum calcium (often > 3.0 mg/dl) to exogenous PTH (200 U) administered im every 8 hrs (up to six doses) and by demonstrating a rise in phosphate excretion and an increase in nephrogenous cyclic AMP in response to intravenous PTH. Unfortunately the usual source of exogenous PTH (extract of bovine parathyroid glands) is no longer commercially available in the United States. The hypocalcemia of idiopathic hypoparathyroidism is severe (the average total serum calcium is 5.4 mg/dl) and requires full doses of calcium and vitamin D.

PSEUDOHYPOPARATHYROIDISM (PHP): PHP is a familial syndrome of hypocalcemia associated with raised levels of PTH and resistance to PTH action. A characteristic physiognomy (Albright's osteodystrophy) of round facies, short stature, and short metacarpals and metatarsals (4th and 5th digits) is present in the classic syndrome. The importance of this syndrome relates not to its frequency but rather to its contribution to our understanding of the pathophysiology of hormone resistance in general. PHP is managed as hypoparathyroidism but is often easier to treat than idiopathic hypoparathyroidism, probably because the hormone resistance is not total. Patients who have the stigmata of Albright's osteodystropy (short stature, obesity, and dystrophic bone changes) without hypocalcemia are said to have pseudopseudohypoparathyroidism (PPHP). PPHP is genetically related but distinct from PHP.

HYPOMAGNESEMIA: Severe hypomagnesemia (under 0.8 meq/l) may caused hypocalcemia by inhibiting PTH effect on bone and by decreasing the secretion of PTH by the parathyroid gland in response to hypocalcemia. This syndrome is found in chronic alcoholism and malabsorption. The hypocalcemia does not respond to calcium loading but is relieved by Mg replacement (page 34).

PANCREATITIS may cause a transitory hypocalcemia. The mechanism remains unexplained.
VITAMIN D DEFICIENCY AND DISORDERS OF VITAMIN D METABOLISM as causes of hypocalcemia are discussed on pages 130-133.

Management of Chronic Hypocalcemia

Chronic hypocalcemia is treated with calcium supplementation and with vitamin D or one of its analogs. Doses in the range of 1.5-2.5 gm of elemental calcium/day are prescribed in divided doses tid. The calcium content of the available preparations varies and one must be certain that the proper amount of elemental calcium is given. Calcium carbonate is the most convenient form since the high calcium content (40%) of this compound means fewer tablets are needed.   Calcium chloride should be avoided because of the high incidence of gastric irritation. The following table lists several calcium preparations, their calcium content, and approximate cost to patient/day for 1.5 gm of elemental calcium.

Table 11.2 Calcium Preparations Used in Treating Hypocalcemia

Compound	Trade Name	Calcium Content	Tabs/Day	Cost/Day*
Calcium Carbonate (tablets)	Os-Cal 500**	500 mg	3	$.40-.50
	Titralac 420 mg	168 mg	9	$.55-.65
	Tums	200 mg	7-8	$.30-.40
Calcium Lactate	Generic 625 mg	80 mg	19	$.85-.90
Calcium Gluconate	Generic 1 gm	90 mg	17	$1.60
Calcium Glubionate	Neo-Calglucon Syrup 5 ml	115 mg	4 tablsp.	$1.40

* Retail cost as of Sept 1983; ** Other forms of Os Cal contain additional drugs and should be avoided.

Vitamin D and its analogs promote intestinal absorption of calcium. The preparation and dose of vitamin D used will vary depending on the underlying cause of the hypocalcemia. Vitamin D2 (ergocalciferol) is the traditional preparation. Its principal advantage is low cost, an important factor to consider since this is a life-time medication for most patients.   D2's disadvantage is that the therapeutic dose is close to the toxic dose and, thus, may cause hypercalcemia. Since this vitamin is stored in fat, it may take up to three months for hypercalcemia to resolve. The onset of action likewise is delayed and may take up to 1-2 months to achieve maximal effect.   Large doses (ergocalciferol 50,000

- 100,000 U/day) are needed for most hypocalcemic disorders since in order to override the relative deficiency of kidney hydroxylase caused by the lack of PTH. Despite these drawbacks, most patients can be managed sucessfully with this preparation. Care is taken to check the serum calcium every 6 months since some patients who appear to be under optimal control will unexpectedly develop hypercalcemia. Smaller doses of ergocalciferol are used to treat vitamin D deficiency (5000 U/day initially, then 400 U/day) and for the anticonvulsant therapy-related hypocalcemia (5000 U/day). Dihydrotachysterol (DHT) is another vitamin D preparation used in the treatment of chronic hypocalcemia. It is a synthetic analog of vitamin D which does not require 1-alpha-hydroxlation by the kidney. The potency of DHT is not as great nor the onset of action as short as the newest vitamin D preparation, 1,25-dihydroxyvitamin D (calcitriol). Calcitriol has the advantages of a rapid onset of action (2-4 days) and a short half-life (12-24 hrs) which allows quick resolution should the complication of hypercalcemia arise. Both DHT and calcitriol offer the theoretical advantage of circumventing the need for renal hydroxylation which is impaired in PTH deficiency and PTH resistance. Cost is the major disadvantage of long-term calcitriol therapy. Calcidiol (25-hydroxyvitamin D) offers no advantages in the treatment of hypocalcemia. The following table lists the preparations of vitamin D and its derivatives.

Table 11.3 Vitamin D Preparations Used to Treat Hypocalcemia

Drug	Trade Name	Dose	Approximate Cost/100 tabs*	Cost/day
Vitamin D2	Drisdol	50,000 U	$19.10	$0.19-0.38
Dihydrotachysterol	Hytakerol	125 ug	$24.00	$0.24-0.96
25-hydroxyvitamin D	Calderol	50 ug	$64.00	$0.64-2.56
1,25-dihydroxy- vitamin D	Rocaltrol	0.25 ug 0.50 ug	$58.00 $96.00	$1.16-6.96 $0.96-5.76

* Retail cost as of Sept 1983; markup may vary up to 50% more.

Those patients with chronic hypocalcemia who require calcium supplementation and vitamin D replacement need to wear proper identification as to their medical diagnosis (e.g., Medic-Alert).

References

Arnaud CD, Clark OH: Primary hyperparathyroidism, in Krieger DT, Bardin CW (eds): Current Therapy in Endocrinology 1983-1984. Burlington, Ontario, BC Decker, 1983, pp 277-282.

Breslau NA, Pak CYC: Hypoparathyroidism. Metabolism 28:1261, 1979.

Broadus AE: Mineral metabolism, in Felig P, Baxter JD, Broadus AE, Frohman LA (eds): Endocrinology and Metabolism. New York, McGraw-Hill, 1981, pp 963-1079.

Habener JF, Potts JT: Parathyroid physiology and primary hyperparathyroidism, in Avioli LV, Krane SM (eds): Metabolic Bone Disease, vol 2. New York, Academic Press, 1978.

Marx SJ, Speigel AM, Brown EM, Koehler JO et al: Divalent cation metabolism. Familial hypocalciuric hypercalcemia versus typical primary hyperparathyroidism. Am J Med 65:235, 1978.

Nordin BEC, Horsman A, Marshall DH, Simpson M, Waterhouse GM: Calcium requirement and calcium therapy. Clin Orthop Relat Res 140:216, 1979.

Patten BM, Bilezikian JP, Mallette LE, Prince A, Engel WK, Aurbach GD: Neuromuscular disease in primary hyperparathyroidism. Ann Intern Med 80:182, 1974.

Simpson EL, Mundy GR, D'Souza SM, Ibbotson KJ, Bockman R, Jacobs JW: Absence of parathyroid hormone messenger RNA in nonparathyroid tumors associated with hypercalcemia. N Engl J Med 309:325, 1983.

Chapter 12

Metabolic Bone Disease

Metabolic bone disease refers to a variety of disorders which affect bony tissue including osteoporosis, osteomalacia, osteitis fibrosa, renal osteodystropy, and osteitis deformans (Paget's disease of bone). Bone is a dynamic tissue which is constantly undergoing change. Remodeling at bone surfaces is a complex process involving matrix (osteoid) synthesis by osteoblasts, mineralization of the matrix to form mature bone, and eventually resorption of calcified bone by osteoclasts. The process which results in mineralization of the osteoid is poorly understood, but proper amounts of calcium, phosphate, vitamin D metabolites, and a normal collagen matrix are necessary for this process to proceed normally. In addition, local factors such as mechanical stress and coupling factors (proteins which link resorption with formation and vice versa) are involved in the remodeling process. Since bone formation and bone resorption are processes which can be modified by the hormonal and chemical milieu, a variety of different disorders may lead to metabolic bone disease.

Osteoporosis: Osteoporosis is the most common metabolic bone disease. It is an important cause of morbidity and mortality for the elderly. Osteoporotic bone has two characteristic features: decreased bone volume (less mineralized matrix per unit volume) and the bone which is present appears normal (matrix is mineralized normally). Osteoporosis affects all bone but trabecular bone (e.g., vertebrae, femoral head, distal radius) is much more involved than compact or cortical bone (e.g., shafts of long bones). The reduced mineral content can be demonstrated as osteopenia on roentgenographs only after there has been more than 30% decrease in trabecular bone mass. The reduction in trabecular bone mass means that these affected bones are subject to collapse and fracture. The osteoporotic patient usually presents with compression fractures of spinal vertebral bodies, fractures of distal radius, or proximal femur.

The pathogenesis of osteoporosis is multifactorial. Bone mineral content reaches its maximum during the third decade of life. The amount of mineral deposited is dependent on body size (thin, petit frame has less mineral than large frame individuals), sex (female < male), and race (Caucasian < Negro). After the third decade there is a gradual reduction in body mineral content that is accelerated in the menopausal female. Estrogen has a vital role in preservation of mineral mass. Estrogen deficiency is associated with lower serum levels of 1,25-dihydroxy-vitamin D which leads to less intestinal absorption of calcium. Estrogen also inhibits parathyroid hormone (PTH) effect on bone absorption. These factors plus an inadequate dietary intake of calcium by most adult women and possibly less sunlight exposure are thought to be the reasons for the acceleration of mineral loss from the bone. Bone biopsy of osteoporotic patients confirms a multifactorial causation since some patients have increased bone resorption as well as decreased bone formation. The patient who has the greatest risk for developing clinical osteoporosis (that is, fractures related to reduced bone mass) is the white, postmenopausal female who has a petit frame or had a petit frame at age of 20 yrs and now is obese.

Although postmenopausal or senile osteoporosis is the most common and least understood catagory of osteoporosis, there are several endocrine abnormalities associated with osteoporosis. These include estrogen deficiency during the premenopausal years as in ovarian dysgenesis (Turner's syndrome) or premature menopause (surgical or idiopathic); testosterone deficiency; Cushing's syndrome; hyper-thyroidism; and primary hyperparathyroidism. Whether diabetes mellitus increases risk of osteoporosis is controversial. Immobilization or weightlessness can also cause osteoporosis.

The clinical presentation of osteoporosis is pain and deformity related to fracture. Back pain is usually the symptom which brings the patient to the physician. The onset of pain may be sudden, aggravated by movement and weight bearing, and relieved by rest. Thoracic and lumbar vertebrate are most affected (especially T12 and L1). Falling is particularly likely to lead to femoral neck fractures or Colles' fracture of the wrist (both areas of considerable trabecular bone). Lost of vertebral height and anterior wedging of the vertebrae lead to shortening of stature and kyphosis.

Laboratory findings are usually not specific with serum Ca, P, and alkaline phosphatase activity being normal. The X-ray will show osteopenia of other areas as well as site of fracture. Ballooning of nuclei pulposi into weakened trabecular bone leads to concave deformities ("codfishing") of the vertebra and localized herniation of the pulposus leads to Schmorl's node.

If there is no generalized osteopenia or if there are serum calcium or phosphatase abnormalities in a female who presents with a compression vertebral fracture, one should consider the possibility of a pathological fracture due to metastatic disease. If there is anemia and vertebral fractures, myeloma should be excluded.

Treatment of newly diagnosed vertebral fractures includes bedrest, analgesics for pain, and local heat for relief of paravertebral muscle spasm which often may develop as the major component of chronic back pain. Avoid using narcotics for analgesia if possible. Early ambulation is recommended. If pain persists, back support in the form of a back brace is used. Patients are cautioned not to lift heavy objects, and to bend at the knees instead of the waist when lifting objects. Exercise such as long walks and swimming is encouraged.

Unfortunately there are no drugs which can provoke or increase the amount of normal bone mass as needed for the treatment of osteoporosis. At present, all medications are given to retard the progression of the loss of mineral mass that accompanies aging. It is difficult to evaluate whether a treatment regimen is suitable or is working in an individual patient since our methods of quantitating bone mass are not very precise. Most recommended treatments are derived from epidemiological studies of populations of patients treated with different regimens. Photon absorption of the radius does not tell anything about the axial skeleton where the loss of mineral is the greatest. Computerized tomography (CT) of the vertebral body has the potential to be useful in following the treatment of osteoporosis.

The safest medication is calcium supplementation 1.0 to 1.5 gm of elemental calcium/day taken as calcium carbonate for convenience (see table 11.2, page 123 for list of calcium preparations). Oral calcium ingestion corrects any negative calcium balance and inhibits bone loss via resorption. It is as effective as any therapy in reducing height loss in patients who have crushed vertebra (fig. 12.1).

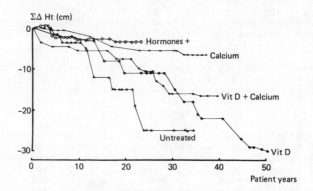

Figure 12.1 The loss of height was reduced with oral calcium (1.5 gm/day) to 0.1 cm/yr in postmenopausal patients with vertebral fractures compared to 0.7 cm/yr for patients with vertebral fractures who received no therapy [Nordin BEC, Horsman A, Marshall DH, Simpson M, Waterhouse GM: Calcium requirement and calcium therapy. <u>Clin Orthop Relat Res</u> 140:216, 1979. with permission].

Estrogen is effective in treating osteoporosis. It retards bone loss by inhibiting PTH-induced resorption and increasing gut absorption of calcium. Estrogen therapy has been demonstrated to reduce the fracture rate in osteoporosis, to reduce the loss of statural height (fig. 12.1), and to retard mineral loss from vertebral bodies as assessed by CT. At least 0.625 mg of conjugated estrogens (e.g., Premarin 0.625 mg/day) are necessary to be effective. However estrogens do have troublesome side effects including vaginal bleeding, increased risk of endometrial carcinoma, and tendency to fluid retention. Using a progestin (e.g., Provera 10 mg q d for 5-10 days every third month on day 20-30) will produce withdrawal uterine bleeding and may decrease the risk of uterine cancer. Annual pelvic and breast exams are necessary and all abnormal vaginal bleeding needs to be promptly investigated. <u>The ideal candidate for estrogen therapy is the woman who has had a hysterectomy.</u>

Vitamin D is not used alone for therapy and is only occasionally used with oral calcium. Providing most patients with small doses of vitamin D2 (400 U/day) is sufficient to meet the D requirements. High doses of vitamin D2 (Drisdal 50,000 U twice a week) can lead to hypercalciuria and possibly to hypercalcemia. As seen in figure 12.1, vitamin D alone does not reduce height loss on osteoporosis.

However, pharmacological doses of vitamin D are used for patients with impaired bowel absorption of calcium. Generally these patients will have < 50 mg of urine calcium/24 hr (normal 200-300 mg/day). These patients may well have osteomalacia in addition to osteoporosis on bone biopsy.

Fluoride increases bone mass but the bone is not normal. The doses used, 40-60 mg/day, are doses which also cause osteomalacia and secondary hyperparathyroidism. Fluoride therapy is still experimental and is not approved for use by the FDA for treatment of osteoporosis.

All patients with osteoporosis are treated with oral calcium 1.5 gm/day. If there are no contra-indications and the patient is perimenopausal, oral estrogen (taken cyclically as conjugated estrogen 0.625 mg days 1-25 with oral progestin added q 3 months) is prescribed. For the patients who have had a hysterectomy, estrogen is taken daily. Exercise is encouraged and immobilization is only for the acute situation. If the response to therapy is poor, reconsider the diagnosis.

If there is a known hormone deficiency such as estrogen deficiency related to surgical oophorectomy, then hormone replacement is indicated. If the osteoporosis relates to glucocorticoid excess, then reduction of steroid if possible is indicated along with oral calcium plus supplemental vitamin D.

Osteomalacia: Osteomalacia is characterized by large amounts of osteoid which do not mineralize. Bone mineralization depends upon adequate concentrations of calcium and phosphorus locally along the surface of normal bone matrix. If the matrix is not mineralized progressively, then large amounts of osteoid accumulate due to the continual formation of matrix by osteoblasts. Again the interrelationships among calcium, phosphate, vitamin D and its metabolites, and parathyroid hormone are important for mineralization of bone. Any disorder which lowers serum calcium or decreases serum phosphate can lead to osteomalacia.

The clinical presentation of osteomalacia depends upon age and severity and duration of the underlying disorder. In children, osteomalacia is called rickets. Rickets causes deformity in areas of bone that are most rapidly growing leading to craniotabes, frontal bossing, enlargement of costochondral junctions ("rachitic rosary"), and bowing of the legs. Large areas of unmineralized and disorganized epiphyseal growth-plate cartilage lead to short stature.

Bone deformity is rare in adult-onset rickets (osteomalacia). What is common in both rickets and osteomalacia is bone pain and local tenderness over severely affected areas. Muscle weakness is common particularly the proximal muscles of the lower extremities. If the patient is also hypocalcemic, paresthesias, tetany, and seizures may be present.

The radiographic picture of advanced childhood rickets is quite characteristic: enlargement of unmineralized epiphyseal growth plates; widening and cupping associated with a frayed appearance of the metaphyses; and pseudofractures. In adults, osteomalacia oftens appears as generalized osteopenia mimicking osteoporosis and making radiographic distinction difficult. A characteristic radiographic feature pathognomonic for osteomalacia is the pseudofracture (Looser zones or Milkman fractures). Pseudofractures are most often bilateral and occur in the femoral neck and shaft, ulna and radius, clavicle, scapula, pubic and ischial rami, and small bones of the hands and feet. Secondary hyperparathyroidism, found in vitamin D deficiency osteomalacia, causes bone resorption manifest by subperiosteal resorption of phalanges, loss of lamina dura of the teeth, resorption of the distal clavicle, widening of the pubic symphysis and the sacroiliac joint space, and bone cysts or brown tumors (see osteitis fibrosa below).

Osteomalacia can be classified biochemically into two subgroups. The first is the result of vitamin D deficiency or altered vitamin D metabolism leading to inadequate calcium absorption from the gut and low serum calcium. Secondary hyperparathyroidism results from the attempt to normalize serum calcium and leads to lowering of the serum phosphorus as a result of PTH-induced phosphaturia. Serum alkaline phosphatase activity is elevated by osteoblastic activation coupled to bone resorption effects of PTH. The second subgroup is related to a defect in phosphate transport leading to phosphaturia and poor gut absorption of phosphorus manifest by normocalcemia and severe hypophosphatemia. The serum alkaline phosphatase activity is also increased. There is no evidence of hyperparathyroidism in this chronic hypophosphatemic group. Assays of vitamin D and its metabolites have been helpful in assessing the heterogeneous causes of osteomalacia. Vitamin D is a prohormone that is eaten in the diet or derived from the conversion of a steroid in the skin to vitamin D by sunlight (UV spectrum). Vitamin D itself has little, if any, biological activity but it is hydroxylated by a liver enzyme, vitamin D 25-hydroxylase, leading to the major vitamin D metabolite in the serum, 25-hydroxyvitamin D. Measurement of serum 25-hydroxyvitamin D is the best indicator of body stores of vitamin D and is low in vitamin

D deficiency states (normal ranges are 8 to 60 ng/ml). The most active metabolite of vitamin D is 1,25-dihydroxyvitamin D which is derived from further hydroxylation of 25-hydroxyvitamin D in the kidney. Elevated PTH levels and low serum phosphorus stimulate the formation of 1,25-dihydroxyvitamin D. Low levels of PTH and high serum phosphorus will lower the level of this metabolite. Normal serum 1,25-dihydroxyvitamin D is 20-50 pg/ml.

Regardless of the causal biochemical defect, the clinical and radiographic presentation of osteomalacia is constant. However, the biochemical defect is helpful in determining the etiology of the osteomalacia and in selecting the most effective therapy. As mentioned above, osteomalacia is classified on the basis of abnormalities related to vitamin D or to chronic hypophosphatemia.

Vitamin D abnormalities include reduced circulating vitamin D metabolites (because of inadequate sunlight exposure, inadequate dietary vitamin D, vitamin D malabsorption as a result of small intestine disease, bile salt or pancreatic insufficiency), and abnormal vitamin D metabolism (due to liver disease, chronic renal failure, drugs such as dilantin and phenobarbital which decrease 25-hydroxyvitamin D levels, mesenchymal tumors and prostatic carcinoma which are associated with low 1,25-dihydroxyvitamin D levels, vitamin-D dependent rickets Type I where the renal 1-alpha hydroxylase activity is very low). Resistance to 1,25-dihydroxyvitamin D is rare and is called vitamin-D dependent rickets Type II.

Vitamin D-related osteomalacia has usually been treated with vitamin D2, the plant-derived vitamin, which is inexpensive. Large enough doses can override many of the above defects by mass action. For prevention of vitamin D deficiency 100 IU/day is sufficient in adults and 400 IU/day for children. Pharmacological doses up to 100,000 IU D2/day are needed in bowel malabsorption osteomalacia. Patients with gluten enteropathy will resolve their osteomalacia with a gluten-free diet alone. Patients taking anticonvulsant therapy need 5000 IU D2/day to treat and prevent osteomalacia. Patients with chronic renal failure and vitamin D-resistant rickets Type I will respond to physiologic amounts of 1,25-dihydroxyvitamin D (0.5-2.0 ug/day).

Each vitamin D preparation has advantages and disadvantages. D2 is cheap and usually effective but the therapeutic dose approaches the toxic dose, the onset of action slow (weeks), and duration is prolonged since this vitamin is stored in fat. Other preparations are available (25-hydroxyvitamin D and dihydrotachysterol) but these are relatively expensive and offer no real practical advantages (see table 11.3, page 124). Calcitriol (1,25-dihydroxy-vitamin D; Rocaltrol) is expensive ($60-70/100 0.25 ug tabs) but the onset of action is rapid (2-4 days) and half-life short (12 hrs). Since calcitriol is thought to be the active compound, no transformation is needed to make it active.

Hypophosphatemic vitamin D-resistant rickets is the most common form of osteomalacia in the United States. Renal phosphate wasting (phosphate diabetes) is the cardinal feature. PTH does not contribute to the phosphaturia. Familial X-linked hypophosphatemic rickets is another name for this syndrome, but the pattern of inheritance is not well established since sporadic and autosomal recessive patterns have been reported. Other maladies associated with significant phosphaturia include Fanconi syndrome and tumor-induced osteomalacia (mesenchymal and prostatic cancer). Chronic hypophosphatemia secondary to phosphate-binding antacids may rarely lead to osteomalacia.

Hypophosphatemic vitamin-D resistant rickets is treated with oral phosphate (elemental P 1-4 gm/day) given in divided doses to minimize diarrhea. Although oral phosphate may raise the serum phosphorus and improve the osteomalacia as assessed by roentgenographs, complete bone healing is seen only in patients treated with phosphates and 1,25-dihydroxyvitamin D, 1-3 ug/day.

Osteitis fibrosa: Osteitis fibrosa is characterized by resorption of bone, osteoclastic activation with focal eroded areas (Howship's lacunae), reactive fibrosis, cyst formation, and brown tumors. Hyperparathyroidism is the underlying biochemical defect causing the bone resorption and subsequent hypercalcemia. 1,25-Dihydroxyvitamin D levels are usually elevated since PTH stimulates the renal synthesis of this metabolite. As a result of coupling reaction in bone, osteoblasts are activated leading to raised levels of alkaline phosphatase activity. Secondary hyperparathyroidism, as in chronic renal failure, may lead to osteitis fibrosa.

The radiographic changes associated with hyper-parathyroidism reflect bone resorption: osteopenia; subperiosteal resorption of phalanges (especially lateral midshaft) and clavicles (particularly lateral ends); and small punched-out lesions of the skull. Osteitis fibrosa cystica represents a late effect of chronic hyperparathyroidism. These classic bone changes are not seen as frequently as in the past since hypercalcemia is often found with screening chemistries.

The treatment of primary hyperparathyroidism is surgery. Removal of the abnormal parathyroid gland(s) is the only real therapy. Estrogens block PTH's effect on bone and should be considered second line treatment. Postoperative hypocalcemia after parathyroid surgery should be anticipated due to the "hungry bone" and treated with oral or iv calcium (page 34).

Renal Osteodystrophy: Renal osteodystrophy is the metabolic bone disease that accompanies chronic renal insufficiency and failure. The combination of hyperphosphatemia (inhibits 1,25-dihydroxyvitamin D synthesis) and loss of renal mass (decreases 25-hydroxyvitamin D 1-alpha hydroxylase) reduces the active D metabolite leading to calcium malabsorption and consequent hypocalcemia. Hypocalcemia leads to osteomalacia as well as secondary hyperparathyroidism. The bone lesions of renal osteodystrophy are highly variable and may reflect osteomalacia or osteitis fibrosa or both. Pain, weakness, and fractures are common with this disorder.

The best treatment of this disorder is prevention since most, if not all, patients with chronic azotemia will develop some form of renal osteodystrophy. Maintenance of normal serum calcium and phosphorus concentrations is the first goal. Restricting dietary phosphorus to 1 gm/day, using phosphate-binding antacids, providing at least 1 to 1.5 gm of elemental calcium/day, and maintaining acid-balance with judicious use of alkali are important therapeutic points in prevention of renal osteodystrophy. Prophylactic use of calcitriol is useful but close follow-up is needed to avoid hypercalcemia and extraskeletal calcification. Bone biospy after tetracycline labelling of the mineralization front (a technique available in centers that evaluate bone histomorphology with UV microscopy) is helpful in patients with advanced bone disease to assess whether there is low turnover osteomalacia or aggressive osteitis fibrosa or combination thereof. Selective partial parathyroidectomy may be necessary for osteitis fibrosa.

Paget's Disease of the Bone (osteitis deformans): Paget's disease is a chronic, patchy and scattered disease affecting localized areas of bone. It is common disease found in up to 4% of the population of Anglo-Saxon origin over the age of forty. The etiology is unknown. The disease may affect one or multiple areas of bone (polyostotic form). The areas of affected bone are characterized by localized osteolysis with giant osteoclasts containing up to 100 nuclei. The number of nuclei within the pagetic osteoclast is much greater than in other metabolic bone diseases. In addition, large numbers of osteoblasts are present forming bone in areas of previous osteolytic activity. Unfortunately this bone structure and modeling is not normal. If severe, these lesions lead to bone deformity and enlargement. Inclusions that have the appearance of viral nucleocapsids have been identified and have raised again the view of Sir James Paget that this disease is inflammatory in nature.

The clinical features are variable. Most patients are <u>asymptomatic</u> and the disorder is discovered as the result of screening chemistries <u>(the serum alkaline phosphatase activity being elevated and the serum calcium and phosphorus being normal.)</u> Chance finding of lytic and sclerotic areas of bone with bone expansion on radiographic examinations is also a frequent method of detecting asymptomatic disease.

Pain and deformity are the most common symptoms. However bone pain doesn't correlate well with the degree of skeletal involvement. Nerve root compression (e.g., acoustic nerve), spinal cord or brainstem compression due to expansive bone, and pathologic fractures in weight-bearing bones are the most severe complications. With the great degree of resorptive and osteoblastic activity, blood flow to the affected bones is greatly increased, leading to increased warmth over these areas. When more than a third of the skeleton is involved, then high output heart failure is possible. The pelvic bone is most frequently involved followed by the femur, skull, tibia, and spine. Lytic and sclerotic areas of bone with bone expansion are seen on roentgenographs. Occult disease not seen on routine X-rays may be demonstrated with radionuclide bone scans.

<u>No treatment is needed for the asymptomatic patient.</u> Non-narcotic analgesics will take care of most of the affected patients. In those with <u>unrelieved pain or those with the complications</u> mentioned above, treatment with either <u>calcitonin or diphosphonates</u> is indicated. The decision as to when to institute therapy and which one of these agents requires clinical discernment. Since these agents have been used for only a decade, pros and cons for each are still evolving.

<u>Calcitonin</u> inhibits bone resorption. Subcutaneous salmon calcitonin 50 to 100 U is given daily until symptoms improve (usually 2-6 weeks later). Thereafter, calcitonin is given three times/week and continued for an undefined period of time (avg 22 months). Alkaline phosphatase activity decreases by 50% after 3 months. Calcitonin is relatively expensive and antibodies to this agent often develop with one fourth of the patients becoming resistant to salmon calcitonin after an initial biochemical remission.

<u>Diphosphonates</u> inhibit both bone resorption and mineralization. Disodium etidronate (Didronil) 5 mg/kg is taken orally daily. Larger doses may be needed but the

risks of mineralization defect (osteomalacia) are greater. The clinical and biochemical response is similar to calcitonin with a few notable exceptions; there is a paradoxical increase in pain in 10% of the patients treated with diphosphonates and radiographic evidence of healing is seldom seen after diphosphonate therapy. Six months of therapy is often followed by a prolonged biochemical remission (1 or more yrs). If symptoms recur, another 6-month course can be instituted.

Another agent that inhibits bone resorption is mithramycin. Although effective, mithramycin is not approved in the U.S. for use in Paget's disease (only for treatment of cancer or hypercalcemia).

Hypercalcemia is generally not seen in ambulatory patients with Paget's disease. However, hypercalcemia may be a considerable problem in the immobilized pagetic patient emphasizing the importance of ambulation and adequate hydration in these patients.

A review the biochemical data of these forms of metabolic bone disease is presented below:

Table 12.1 Summary of the Biochemical Data in Metabolic Bone Disease

Bone Disorder	Serum Calcium	Serum Phosphorus	Alkaline Phosphatase	Urine Calcium
Osteoporosis	normal	normal	normal	normal*
Osteomalacia	low**	very low	high	low
Osteitis fibrosa	high	low	high	high
Renal Osteodystrophy	low	high	high	low
Paget's Disease	normal	normal	very high	normal

   * usually normal but may be high (immobilization)
        or low (poor calcium intake)
  ** low in vitamin D abnormalities but low normal
        in chronic hypophosphatemic rickets

References

Avioli LV: Osteoporosis: pathogenesis and therapy, in Avioli LV, Krane SM (eds): Metabolic Bone Disease. New York, Academic Press, 1977, pp 307-385.

Bell NH: Rickets, in Krieger DT, Bardin CW (eds): Current Therapy in Endocrinology 1983-1984. Burlington, Ontario, BC Decker, 1983, pp 245-250.

Hahn TJ: Drug-induced disorders of vitamin D and mineral metabolism. Clin Endocrinol Metabol 9:107, 1980.

Marel GM, Frame B: Osteomalacia, in Krieger DT, Bardin CW (eds): Current Therapy in Endocrinology 1983-1984. Burlington, Ontario, BC Decker, 1983, pp 250-259.

Nordin BEC, Horsman A, Marshall DH, Simpson M, Waterhouse GM: Calcium requirement and calcium therapy. Clin Orthop Relat Res 140:216, 1979.

Singer FR: Metabolic Bone Disease, in Felig P, Baxter JD, Broadus AE, Frohman LA: Endocrinology and Metabolism. New York, McGraw-Hill, 1981, pp 1081-1118.

Chapter 13

Adrenal Disease

Disorders of the adrenal glands are uncommon. However many of the classic symptoms and signs of adrenal diseases mimic those of some common medical disorders such as hypertension, obesity, anxiety, depression, and diabetes mellitus. Thus, adrenal disorders are frequently considered whenever these conditions are encountered since correction of any underlying adrenal disease will often cure the "common" medical disorder.

The adrenal cortex secretes cortisol (the principal glucocorticoid), aldosterone (the primary mineralo-corticoid), and dehydroeipandrosterone and androstenedione (the predominant androgens). The adrenal medulla secretes the catecholamines epinephrine and norepinephrine. Disorders of these adrenal hormones are discussed in the following paragraphs.

GLUCOCORTICOID EXCESS:

The most common cause of Cushing's syndrome is the use of pharmacologic doses of potent glucocorticoids for non-endocrine disorders. There are three endogenous causes of Cushing's syndrome: 1) Cushing's disease (pituitary-dependent adrenal hyperplasia) which represents 70-80% of all cases of Cushing's syndrome; 2) ectopic ACTH syndrome (ACTH secreted by non-pituitary tumors); and 3) adrenal tumors (adenoma or carcinoma).

The clinical manifestations of glucocorticoid excess are identical with the first and third causes whereas the second cause (ectopic ACTH syndrome) usually has few of the chronic changes induced by excess glucocorticoids (e.g., obesity, osteoporosis, etc.) and more of the biochemical changes associated with high doses of corticoids (e.g., hypokalemia and metabolic alkalosis).

The clinical features of endogenous Cushing's syndrome are due to the combined effect of glucocorticoids, mineralocorticoids, and adrenal androgens. Obesity is the most common feature with the deposition of adipose tissue especially in the face (round facies) and under the chin (dewlap), on the dorsal and supraclavicular fat pads, and over the trunk and abdomen. This gives a characteristic physique, vis-à-vis, truncal obesity. This centripetal obesity is accentuated by wasting of the extremities caused by the catabolic effect of excess glucocorticoids on muscle protein metabolism. The skin is thin and paperlike, producing facial plethora and less frequently violaceous striae. Protein catabolism leads to muscle weakness, back pain due to osteoporosis, and easy bruising. Hypertension is virtually universal in patients over 40 yrs of age (reflecting excess mineralocorticoid activity) but much less common in younger patients. Mild hirsutism, menstrual disorders, and acne are the result of excess adrenal androgens. Psychological disturbances are present in 2/3 of Cushing's patients and may be dramatic with severe depression, psychosis, or mania. Fasting hyperglycemia is found in 10-15% of the patients. Hypokalemia and metabolic alkalosis is characteristic of ectopic ACTH syndrome.

Workup of Cushing's Syndrome

The general appearance of the patient often leads one to suspect glucocorticoid excess. Serial photographs taken months and years earlier are most informative (start with driver's license or employment photo). Is the patient taking medication? Always search for a pharmaceutical source of steroids. Is the patient a female? Cushing's disease is ten times more common in females than males. What is the age of the patient? Cushing's disease is most frequent in ages 20-40 yrs. Ectopic ACTH syndrome is generally a disease of the older population. Is there weight loss to suggest ectopic ACTH? Oat cell carcinoma of the lung causes at least half the cases of ectopic ACTH production. Other tumors that secrete ACTH include pancreatic islet cell carcinoma, thymoma, carcinoid tumors, medullary thyroid carcinoma, and pheochromocytoma.

A 24-hr urine cortisol should be measured in all suspected cases. Serum cortisol determinations are not very helpful unless coupled with dexamethasone testing (page 12). If the urine cortisol is increased, then several dynamic studies are available to identify the source of the hypercortisolism (pages 12-13). ACTH determinations can be helpful if locally available. Very high levels are found in ectopic ACTH syndromes and nonmeasurable ACTH levels with adrenal tumors. Very elevated urinary 17-ketosteroids (higher than the urinary 17-OHCS) suggest adrenal carcinoma. Hypokalemia and metabolic alkalosis in the absence of diuretic therapy suggests ectopic ACTH as does a chest X-ray demonstrating a mass lesion.

The best radiographic study to localize the etiology of the Cushing's syndrome is the high resolution CT scan. Adrenal tumors can be identified with the adrenal CT scan. Unfortunately the CT scan of the pituitary is not diagnostic in many patients with Cushing's disease. The rare patient in whom Cushing's disease cannot be differentiated from ectopic ACTH (e.g., particularly that caused by indolent carcinoid tumors) may need catheterization of the inferior petrosal sinuses (venous drainage of the anterior pituitary) to measure ACTH gradients and identify the pituitary as the source of ACTH.

Treatment of Cushing's Syndrome: The treatment of Cushing's disease has already been discussed (page 65). The treatment of adrenal adenoma or carcinoma is by surgical adrenalectomy and even nephrectomy for the large and invasive adrenal carcinoma. Since removal of the tumor causing ectopic ACTH syndrome is rarely possible, treatment of the hypercortisolism with inhibitors of cortisol biosynthesis will help the weakness and hyperkalemia. Two adrenal enzyme inhibitors are available for blocking steriodogenesis: aminoglutethimide and metyrapone. Aminoglutethimide (250 mg qid) or metyrapone (250-500 mg qid) decreases cortisol production and replacement glucocorticoids are not usually needed. O,p'DDD is used to treat adrenal carcinoma that can not be totally removed and for metastatic adrenal carcinoma. Metastatic adrenal carcinoma has a poor prognosis with < 50% survival at three yrs despite o,p'DDD therapy.

ADRENOCORTICAL INSUFFICIENCY:

Inadequate adrenal function results from destruction of the cortex (primary adrenal insufficiency or Addison's disease) or from adrenocortical atrophy due to ACTH deficiency (secondary adrenal insufficiency). In this latter circumstance mineralocorticoid function is preserved since the predominant regulator of aldosterone synthesis is the renin-angiotensin system not ACTH. There must be > 90% destruction of the adrenal gland before Addison's disease is clinically apparent.

Eighty per cent of Addison's disease is caused by autoimmune destruction of the adrenal glands which is sometimes associated with other forms of polyglandular failure. Other causes of adrenal failure include granulomatous diseases (tuberculosis, histoplasmosis, sarcoidosis) and rarely infiltrative diseases (amyloid, lymphoma, hemochromatosis, and metastatic disease). One cause of adrenal insufficiency to be considered whenever a patient is taking anticoagulant medication is bilateral adrenal hemorrhage. This usually occurs within 7-10 days after therapy is started and is associated with back pain.

Secondary adrenal atrophy due to hypopituitarism has already been discussed (pages 66-68). Exogenous glucocorticoids cause adrenal atrophy via suppression of ACTH. The same mechanism produces contralateral adrenal atrophy in cases of adrenal tumor causing Cushing's syndrome.

Clinical features of chronic adrenal insufficiency include: <u>weakness, fatigue, and anorexia</u> which are invariably present and <u>gastrointestinal complaints</u> of nausea, vague abdominal pain, and vomiting which are seen less frequently. Salt craving is present in 20% of patients. Physical findings of <u>weight loss, hyper-pigmentation, and hypotension</u> are generally found. The increased pigmentation results from increased melanin stimulation associated with raised ACTH levels. The hyperpigmentation is generalized but is accentuated in sun-exposed areas, the scrotum and perineum, nipple areola, skin creases, and areas subject to repeated trauma such as elbows, knuckles, and knees. These skin changes are not present in secondary adrenal insufficiency. Some Addisonian patients have stone-hard pinna caused by calcification of the auricular cartilage.

Low AM serum cortisol and elevated plasma ACTH are the diagnostic laboratory findings of Addison's disease. The cortisol does not rise following ACTH administration (page 18). Mineralocorticoid deficiency is manifest as <u>hyponatremia and hyperkalemia.</u> The BUN is elevated reflecting the prerenal azotemia of salt wasting and volume contraction. Hypercalcemia is present in 6% cases of Addison's disease and remits with therapy. Fasting hypoglycemia may occur especially during crisis situations because of lack of glucocorticoid effect. Adrenal crisis may be precipated by any stress situation including fever, infection, radiographic studies, surgery, etc. (page 27). A normochromic and normocytic anemia associated with an eosinophilia is commonly present. If a macrocytic anemia is present, one should suspect concomitant pernicious anemia.

Workup of the Hypoadrenal Patient

Once the diagnosis of hypoadrenalism is considered it is not difficult to exclude or confirm. Any patient with unexplained weight loss should be suspect for Addison's disease (other endocrine diseases to be considered are thyrotoxicosis and diabetes mellitus). Are there symptoms compatible with hypoadrenalism (weakness, nausea, anorexia, etc.)? Has the patient suddenly stopped taking glucocorticoids? Is there a precipitating cause that has unmasked insufficient adrenal reserve? <u>Is there hyperpigmentation?</u> Often the Addisonian patient will present in adrenal crisis with hypotension, hypovolemia, abdominal pain which may mimic an acute abdomen, and possibly fever. A tip-off to adrenal insufficiency may come from the determination of serum cortisol during stress. Any subject with normal adrenal glands will have serum cortisol levels > 20 ug/dl during severe stress. Finding hyponatremia, hyperkalemia, and azotemia should suggest the possibility of hypoadrenalism. If the diagnosis of hypoadrenalism is suspected during a stress situation, one should obtain blood for cortisol and ACTH determinations and immediately begin Solu-Cortef iv along with normal saline as discussed on page 28. If the diagnosis is suspected in a non-acute situation or seems less likely, then provocative testing with a short course of ACTH is indicated (page 18).

Treatment of Adrenal Insufficiency: The treatment for adrenal crisis is discussed on page 28. The management during stress such as preparation for and during surgery is described on pages 70-71. In the non-stressed situation, the euadrenal state is maintained with hydrocortisone (cortisol) 20-30 mg/day usually given bid 10-20 mg at 7-8 AM and 10 mg at 4-6 PM. An occasional patient may need 10 mg tid. Hydrocortisone is rapidly absorbed from the gut and serum levels of cortisol peak after about 1 hr. Cortisone acetate may also be used for replacement. The dose is 25-37.5 mg/day given as 12.5-25 mg q AM and 12.5 mg q PM identical to the hydrocortisone schelude. Cortisone acetate is absorbed just slightly more slowly than hydrocortisone and is converted to cortisol by numerous tissues. In recent years cortisone acetate has cost more than hydrocortisone. Since the half-life of cortisol is 60-90 minutes, the serum cortisol falls to < 3 ug/dl in the Addisonian patient 6-7 hrs after ingesting replacement doses. To evaluate whether replacement dosage is adequate, the clinician must assess the patient for signs and symptoms of inadequate or excessive steroid replacement. Measurement of urine cortisol in patients on replacement is helpful in assuring proper doses of either hydrocortisone or cortisone acetate. Patients with hypopituitary hypoadrenalism need only glucocorticoid replacement since the renin-angiotensin system, which is the predominant regulator of mineralocorticoid metabolism, remains intact. On the other hand, most patients with primary adrenal insufficiency will need mineralocorticoid supplementation although some patients will do well on glucocorticoid therapy alone with liberal salt intake. Fludrocortisone (Florinef) is the mineralocorticoid preparation of choice because it is potent, has prolonged activity, and is less expensive than aldosterone or deoxycorticosterone. The dose of Florinef is 0.05-0.1 mg given as a single dose once a day or every other day as needed.

Infants and young children with adrenal insufficiency may present with failure to thrive, dehydration and salt wasting, and ambiguous genitalia in the female with masculinization. Decreased activity of one of several adrenal enzymes leads to impaired cortisol production. As a result, ACTH secretion increases and the adrenal enlarges, hence, the name of <u>congenital adrenal hyperplasia.</u> Precursor steroids are shunted along accessory metabolic pathways leading to excessive androgen production (21-hydroxylase and 11-hydroxylase deficiency) and mineralocorticoid production (11-hydroxylase deficiency).

<u>Hyperandrogenism</u> as it relates to hirsutism is discussed on page 88.

<u>HYPERALDOSTERONISM:</u>

Excessive aldosterone production by autonomous functioning adrenal tissue (either an <u>adenoma or hypertrophied zona glomerulosa)</u> stimulates renal wasting of potassium and reabsorption of sodium. The clinical features of hyperaldosteronism reflect <u>volume expansion which leads to hypertension and hypokalemia.</u> Hyperaldosteronism is a rare cause of hypertension (much less than 1%). The key to the diagnosis is a suspicion of its possibility in any <u>hypokalemic hypertensive patient who is not taking diuretics.</u> The hypertension can be cured by surgery if an aldosterone-secreting adrenal adenoma is present. Aldosteronoma is more common in females (70% of the cases) whereas bilateral adrenal hypertrophy is seen with equal frequency in both sexes. Unfortunately hypertension caused by bilateral adrenal hypertrophy does not respond to adrenalectomy.

<u>Most hyperaldosteronism is secondary,</u> i.e., reflecting a normal adrenal response to increased stimulation by the renin-angiotensin system. A decrease in effective blood volume (e.g., diuretic therapy, hepatic insufficiency, congestive heart failure, or nephrotic syndrome) or a decrease in renal perfusion (e.g., malignant hypertension or renal artery stenosis) stimulates renin production and angiotensin generation leading to secondary hyperaldosteronism.

Workup of Hyperaldosteronism

Any patient with hypertension and hypokalemia who is not taking diuretics needs to be evaluated for hyperaldosteronism. The symptoms are non-specific and are related to hypokalemia: weakness, fatigue, and malaise. A history of medication use is important. Excessive ingestion of licorice (glycyrrhizinic acid found in licorice has mineralocorticoid activity) mimics hyperaldosteronism. Patients who chew tobacco that is heavily flavored with licorice may present with hypertension and hypokalemia. The plasma renin activity and urine aldosterone is low in these patients. Edema is absent in primary aldosteronism but is often present in secondary aldosteronism.

One should suspect hyperaldosteronism (primary or secondary) when there is hypokalemia and urinary potassium wasting (> 50 meq/24hrs). Almost all patients with primary aldosteronism will have serum potassium < 4 meq/l. With sodium intake restriction, hypokalemia and urine potassium wasting may be not be present. The diagnosis of primary aldosteronism is made by demonstrating that renin-angiotensin is suppressed and that urine aldosterone is elevated in the face of adequate sodium repletion. A normal or elevated plasma renin activity excludes primary hyperaldosteronism. A low plasma renin does not in itself make the diagnosis since 15-20% of the hypertensive population have suppressed renin activity. Thus, hypokalemia and low renin activity require that a 24-hr urine for aldosterone be collected. If the urine aldosterone is elevated then one must determine whether the cause of the hyperaldosteronism is an adrenal adenoma or bilateral adrenal hyperplasia. Localization with a high resolution CT scan is extremely helpful. If the CT is positive for an adrenal mass, then surgery to remove the adenoma is required. If the CT scan is not diagnostic, then studies measuring plasma aldosterone response to posture are indicated (page 19). Since patients with bilateral hyperplasia retain some responsiveness of the renin-angiotensin system, these patients will raise plasma aldosterone in response to erect posture following overnight recumbency; patients with adenoma have no such response. Plasma aldosterone is measured while recumbent at 8 AM and at 12 noon after spending the morning walking about. If the plasma aldosterone does not rise (value after 4 hrs of upright posture is same as the 8 AM recumbent value) and the CT scan is negative, then venous catheterization of the adrenals may demonstrate gradients of plasma aldosterone which localize the adenoma.

Treatment of aldosteronoma is by surgical removal of the adenoma. Since the hypertension of bilateral hyperplasia responds poorly to surgery and since adrenalectomy leaves these patients dependent on exogenous steroids for remainder of their lives, the treatment of the hyperaldosteronism due to bilateral adrenal hyperplasia is with spironolactone (100-400 mg/day). Spironolactone blocks the renal tubular effect of aldosterone and weakly inhibits aldosterone synthesis. Side effects of spironolactone at > 100 mg/day are common and include gastrointestinal irritation, decreased libido, impotence, menstrual disturbances, and gynecomastia.

HYPOALDOSTERONISM:

Hypoaldosteronism associated with hypocortisolism and salt wasting (Addison's disease) is discussed above. Since the primary regulator of aldosterone secretion is angiotensin II, any deficiency in the renin-angiotensin system may lead to hypoaldosteronism. Hyporeninemic hypoaldosteronism is caused by absent renin production by the kidney and is invariably seen in patients with renal insufficiency. Hyperkalemia and hyperchloremic acidosis along with azotemia are the biochemical findings. More than half the patients have diabetes mellitus. The treatment is with fludrocortisone at higher doses (0.2 mg/day) than are normally required for Addison's disease. Better control of the blood sugar will often ameliorate the hyperkalemia in the diabetic patient.

PHEOCHROMOCYTOMA:

Excessive production of catecholamines by tumors of chromaffin tissue of either the adrenal medulla or extra-adrenal sites will lead to hypertension. The hypertension is sometimes episodic and severe, but sustained hypertension is present in a majority of patients. The clinical features depend upon the predominant catecholamine secreted. Norepinephrine producing tumors are the most common and have hypertension as the primary manifestation. If these tumors also secrete significant amounts of epinephrine then sweating, nervousness, and palpitations are present. A pure epinephrine secreting tumor is rare and is marked by tachycardia, hypertension, and postural hypotension due to epinephrine's effect on the beta-adrenergic receptor causing vasodilation. Headache, excessive perspiration, and palpitations are frequent symptoms of pheochromocytoma. Paroxysmal attacks of such symptoms may be provoked by exercise, postural change, abdominal palpation, urination (chromaffin tissue in the bladder wall is a rare site for tumor), or ingesting some foods while being treated with monoamine oxidase inhibitors (certain cheeses and wines contain tyramine which increases the release of catecholamines).

Workup of Pheochromocytoma

A family history of pheochromocytoma should be sought. Approximately 10% of the cases of pheochromocytoma are familial and occur as simple familial pheochromocytoma or as part of the multiple endocrine neoplasia syndrome (MEN type

IIa or IIb). These patients are younger than the sporadic cases and often have bilateral adrenal and extra-adrenal sites of disease. Neurofibromatosis and cafe-au-lait spots are associated with pheochromocytomas and should be sought by physical exam.

The diagnosis of pheochromocytoma cannot be made on clinical grounds alone. The suspicion of a catecholamine producing tumor is raised in a hypertensive patient who has "spells" of sweating, headache, and palpitation. The diagnosis requires biochemical evidence of increased catecholamine production. A 24-hr urine for catecholamines, metanephrines, or VMA (vanillyl mandelic acid-a catechol breakdown product) should be ordered in such patients (page 19). Often two of these tests are ordered if the index of suspicion is very high to avoid missing the occasional patient that may not have an elevated value on one of these studies. Provocative testing with agents such as tyramine, histamine, or glucagon is not advised because the results are unreliable and the hazards related to the testing are substantial. Localization of pheochromocytoma is facilitated by use of the CT scan. In sporadic cases of pheochromocytoma the adrenal tumor is usually unilateral, but in familial disease these tumors are bilateral and often extra-adrenal. All patients with familial pheochromocytoma should have plasma calcitonin measured to identify the patients with MEN II. This will not affect the immediate therapy of the pheochromocytoma. A chest X-ray should be performed in search of thoracic tumors prior to abdominal surgery.

The treatment of pheochromocytoma is surgical removal. Preoperative management is by alpha adrenergic receptor blockade using phenoxybenzamine (Dibenzyline) in initial dose of 10 mg tid. The dose is increased over several days (up to 40 mg tid) until the blood pressure stabilizes, symptoms abate, and hypovolemia remits. Urine determinations for VMA and metanephrines are not affected by this medication. Propanolol is rarely used and then only after alpha blockade is assured. Intravenous phentolamine (10-20 mg in 250 ml given as a microdrip and titrated to avoid irreversible shock) is used to treat acute hypertension episodes, although nitroprusside is an acceptable alternative. Intraoperative management requires expert anesthesia care. Propranolol and/or lidocaine are used to treat cardiac arrhythmias. The entire abdomen is explored searching for multiple tumors along the aortic chain. Fortunately < 5% of pheochromocytomas are malignant. Patients with metastatic tumor can have their adrenergic symptoms controlled with phenoxybenzamine but there is no effective chemotherapy for malignant pheochromocytoma.

References

Aron DC, Tyrell JB, Fitzgerald PA, Findling JW, Forsham PH: Cushing's syndrome: problems in diagnosis. Medicine 60:24, 1981.

Baxter JD, Tyrell JB: The adrenal cortex, in Felig P, Baxter JD, Broadus AE, Frohman LA (eds): Endocrinology and Metabolism. New York, McGraw-Hill, 1981, pp 385-510.

Burch WM: Urine-free cortisol determination: a useful tool in the management of chronic hypoadrenal states. JAMA 247:2002, 1982.

Crapo L: Cushing's syndrome: a review of diagnostic tests. Metabolism 28:955, 1979.

Cryer PE: Diseases of the adrenal medullae and sympathetic nervous system, in Felig P, Baxter JD, Broadus AE, Frohman LA (eds): Endocrinology and Metabolism. New York, McGraw-Hill, 1981, pp 511-550.

Orth DN: Cushing's syndrome, in Kreiger DT, Bardin CW (eds): Current Therapy in Endocrinology 1983-1984. Burlington, Ontario, BC Decker, 1983, pp 119-127.

Sjoerdsma A, Engelman K, Waldmann TA, Cooperman LH, Hammond WG: Pheochromocytoma: current concepts of diagnosis and treatment. Ann Intern Med 65:1302, 1966.

Weinberger MH, Grim CE, Hollifield JW, et al: Primary aldosteronism: diagnosis, localization, and treatment. Ann Intern Med 90:386, 1979.

Chapter 14

The Weak and Tired Patient

Weakness, tiredness, fatigue, and lack of "energy" are frequent complaints voiced in the clinic or office of any physician. The non-specificity of such complaints opens a Pandora's box of possible diagnoses. To make any sense out of these symptoms, one must integrate them with other symptoms or physical signs. Onset and duration of symptoms, associated pain, weight change, fever, and medications are points which one needs to know. Important differential diagnoses which should be part of the thought process during the interview include anemia, cancer, renal or hepatic insufficency, systemic infection, pulmonary disease, congestive heart failure, arthritides, diabetes mellitus, thyroid disease, and drugs (including alcohol).

Often the clinician must assess whether the tired and weak patient has a "metabolic" problem. This patient may have seen several other physicians seeking help for their fatigue and weakness. Although in most cases the asthenia cannot be attributed to a specific endocrine abnormality, these patients deserve the benefit of an honest attempt to address their problem. It is all too easy to make a premature diagnosis before actually hearing the patient out when she or he presents self-referred for "hypoglycemia" or with "maladie du petit papier." A thorough, unhurried interview and a sympathetic clinician may find a problem missed by others. The importance of an open mind, good history-taking, and complete physical examination can not be overemphasized in dealing with the weak and tired patient.

A logical approach to the weak, tired, dizzy, and gassy patient from the endocrine viewpoint is to ask specific questions that relate to possible hormonal causes. Examples for several hormones and representative questions for each are as follows:

Pituitary: Are menses regular? Regular intervals of menstruation make hypopituitarism unlikely. Is there galactorrhea which may be related to a prolactinoma? Has there been acral growth? Has there been a change in visual acuity? Loss of vision is relatively common with large pituitary tumors.

Adrenal: Is there hyperpigmentation? Chronic primary
adrenal   insufficiency   leads   to   darkening   of   skin
particularly   in   areas   of   repeated   pressure.   Is there
any weight loss, nausea, vomiting or syncope?   Is
there   evidence   of   hypercortisolism?   Episodes   of
tachycardia, headaches, and sweating are suggestive of
pheochromocytoma.

Thyroid: Is   there   a   change   in   neck   size   or   shape   to
suggest   a   goiter?   What   is   the   patient's   room
temperature   preference;   60°,   70°,   or   80°?   If 60°,
this suggests hyperthyroidism; if 80°, then possible
hypothyroidism.   Are there other symptoms and signs of
hypothyroidism   (e.g.,   hoarseness,   muscle   cramps,
sleepiness,   dry skin,   puffy facies,   delayed relaxation
time   of   deep   tendon   reflexes)   or   hyperthyroidism
(e.g., nervousness, anxiety, weight loss despite good
appetite,   increased   sweating,   smooth   skin,   tremor,
proptosis, tachycardia)? Neck pain?

Parathyroid: Has there ever been thyroid or neck
surgery?   Surgical   hypoparathyroidism   is   the   most
common   cause   of   hypocalcemia.   Kidney   stones,
polyuria, and constipation point to hypercalcemia.

Pancreas: Is there nocturia? Noctidipsia? Diabetes
mellitus   with   glycosuria with osmotic diuresis should
considered.   Weight loss despite increased appetite to
go along with diabetes mellitus? Are there symptoms
compatible   with   fasting   hypoglycemia   (e.g.,   mental
confusion,   "glassy"   eyes,   and   sweating   relieved by
food)?

Testes: Is there impotence? Impotence due to primary
hypogonadism is responsive to androgen replacement.

Ovaries: Is   there   premature   menopause?   Is   there
amenorrhea/galactorrhea   compatible   with   a   prolactinoma?

More   often   than   not   the   patient   who   presents   with
weakness   has   chronic fatigue,   is a female between 20 and 50
years   old,   and   many times has the idea that something like
hypoglycemia   "must" be the cause of the weakness and lack of
energy.   The history may be reiterated from a sheet of paper
"so   I   won't   forget   anything."   Social   and   interpersonal
relationships   on   the job and at home with spouse, children,
and   family   members   are   often   a   source   of   unadmitted
conflict.   Anxiety/stress   is the most common diagnosis; yet
this   should be a diagnosis of exclusion made after a careful
review   of   the   history,   physical   exam,   and   laboratory
studies.   Specific   lab   studies   are   warranted   as   deemed

necessary by the history and physical exam and may be needed
to assure the patient that nothing has been overlooked.

Screening laboratory studies using automated techniques
are useful. These include CBC; urine analysis; serum Na, K,
HCO3, Cl, BUN; plasma glucose; serum Ca; serum SGOT, SGPT,
bilirubin, and alkaline phosphatase activity.

Thyroid and adrenal function can be assesed if necessary
as detailed on pages 1-4 and 17-18 respectively.

Although postprandial reactive hypoglycemia probably
exists, it is very difficult to separate this condition from
pseudohypoglycemia or nonhypoglycemia as discussed in the
chapter on HYPOGLYCEMIA (page 53). There is no good test to
used to confirm this "entity". If one orders a oral glucose
tolerance test, then be prepared to defend the results
(either negative or positive) to the patient.

Absent menses in a women of child-bearing years can be
due to pregnancy which must be excluded. Serum prolactin is
obtained when there is a history of amenorrhea or oligomenorrhea and/or galactorrhea.

Serum testosterone and gonadotropins (FSH and LH) are
indicated if hypogonadism is a possibility.

If the clinical index for suspicion of any endocrine
diagnosis is low and the laboratory results do not point to
a specific problem, then be honest with the patient; give
your opinion; but remember the fifteenth century proverb
which summarizes the purpose of medicine:

"To cure sometimes, to relieve often, to comfort always."

This appendix contains information helpful in the care and management of diabetes mellitus. A condensed flow sheet to be used in treating diabetic ketoacidosis is on the following page. A checklist (pages 153 and 154) assures that the patient receives adequate information necessary for optimal care of their diabetes. The last page in the Appendix lists recommendations to the patient so there is no misunderstanding regarding diet, insulin schelude (including dosage adjustments and supplements), and blood or urine monitoring. This sheet and the algorithms for hyperglycemia and hypoglycemia (page 46) are given to the patient.

DIABETIC KETOACIDOSIS FLOW SHEET

PATIENT'S NAME _____
ADMISSION DATE _____

	HOURS POST ADMISSION						
Clock Time	0	2	4	6	8	10	12

CLINICAL:
Weight (q d)
Pulse (q hr)
Respiration (q hr)
Blood Pressure (q h)
Temperature (q 2 hr)
Mental Status (q hr)
ECG (q hr; T wave)

LABORATORY:
Serum:
  Glucose (q 2-4 hr)
  Na (q 4 hr)
  K (q 1-2 hr)
  Cl (q 4 hr)
  HCO3 (q 2-4 hr)
  Acetone (q 4 hr)
  BUN (q 12-24 hr)
  PO4 (q 12-24 hr)
  Mg (q 12-24 hr)
  BUN (q 12-24 hr)

Blood:
  Hgb (q 4-8 hr)
  Hct (q 4-8 hr)
  Art. pH (q 4-12 h)
  Art. CO2 (q 4-12 h)

TREATMENT:

IV Fluids (ml/hr)

Urine Output (ml/hr)

Insulin (U/hr)
Sodium (meq/hr)
Potassium (meq/hr)
Phosphate (mmol/hr)
Bicarbonate (meq/hr)

Diabetes Education Checklist

PHYSICIANS: Check appropiate [ ] for desired instruction and fill in blanks for specific details.

GENERAL INFORMATION:
    [ ] Definition, Incidence, Pathophysiology, Symptoms and Stages
    [ ] Diagnosis: Clues (3 P's), Urine Sugar, Blood Sugar, Tolerance Tests
    [ ] Etiology (heredity, insulin-dependent, insulin resistance)
    [ ] Ketosis-prone vs Ketosis-Resistant Diabetes
    [ ] Effect on Survival
    [ ] Indentification Bracelet or Medallion (e.g., Medic-Alert)
    [ ] Diabetes Association Membership (local meetings, etc.)
    [ ] Literature list: _____

THERAPY:
    [ ] Overall Goals and Objectives
        Diet   Who prepares food? _____
        [ ] Objectives
        [ ] Prescription: Calories _____
                _____ Gms CHO _____ Gms Protein
                How divided? _____ [ ] Polyunsaturates
        [ ] Exchange system
    [ ] Oral Agents   Specific drug? _____ Dose? _____
    [ ] Insulin
        [ ] Objectives
        [ ] Types, actions
        Patient will use _____ Dose? _____
        Administration and care of equipment   [ ] Disposable syringe
        [ ] Glass syringe   [ ] Disposable or [ ] Reusable Needle
        [ ] Storage
        [ ] Rotation of injection sites
        [ ] Mixing insulins
    Therapy Regulation
        [ ] Exercise
        [ ] Acute Illness
        [ ] General glycosuria
        [ ] Hypoglycemia with negative urine
    [ ] Exercise
        [ ] Specific recommendations _____

MONITORING:
    [ ] Purpose, recording results
        Urine glucose (Double-void qualitative)
        [ ] Purpose, threshold
        [ ] Frequency _____
        [ ] Type? Clinitest [ ] 2 drop [ ] 5 drop Tes-tape [ ] Other___
        [ ] Log Book   [ ] Clinilog [ ] Other _____
        Urine ketones
        [ ] Purpose, indications
        [ ] Acetest [ ] Ketostix [ ] Other _____

MONITORING (cont'd):
 Blood Glucose
  [ ] Purpose
  [ ] Reagent Strips (types, cost, storage)
  [ ] Lancets and Automatic Fingerstick Apparatus
  [ ] Frequency _____
  [ ] Reflectometer (Use and standardization)
 Monitoring for Complications
  [ ] Annual physicals
  [ ] Eye exams (particularly after 10 years of onset)
  [ ] Renal function
  [ ] Lipids

COMPLICATIONS:
 Acute
 Ketoacidosis:
  [ ] Pathogenesis, definition
  [ ] Symptoms and diagnosis
  [ ] Therapy: clear liquids [ ] ____ U regular/% urine glucose ac
   [ ] ____ U regular for blood glucose (see Recommendations #6)
 Hypoglycemia:
  [ ] Pathogenesis, definition
  [ ] Symptoms and diagnosis
  [ ] Therapy: 1 fruit exchange ____ Honey or glucose ____
   [ ] Glucagon [ ] Teach technique to family
  [ ] Visual (blurry until blood glucose stabilizes)
 Chronic [ ] Relation to control [ ] Neuropathy [ ] Nephropathy
  [ ] Retinopathy [ ] Vascular [ ] Dermopathy [ ] Infections

General Care:
  [ ] Avoid temperature extremes, harsh antiseptics
  [ ] Foot care and inspection (toenails, calluses, corns, etc.)
 When to call doctor:
  [ ] urine >____% + ketones
  [ ] blood sugar >_____ mg/dl + ketones
  [ ] hypoglycemia [ ] hypoglycemia + heavy spills the same day
  [ ] inability to retain food
  [ ] ulcer or infections
  [ ] other _____
  [ ] Physician's telephone #_____
  [ ] Pregnancy

Report of Instructors: Comment as to comprehension (none, vague,
incomplete, or complete). Note specific areas where there are problems
and where repeated instructions are necessary.

_____
_____
_____

Signed _____, Title. _____, Title.
Date _____

RECOMMENDATIONS FOR DIABETES MANAGEMENT

1) Recommended MEAL PLAN:

_____

2) Prescribed INSULIN dosage:

   MORNING _____

   AFTERNOON _____
Take morning insulin 30 to 60 minutes before breakfast and afternoon
insulin 30 to 60 minutes before the evening meal.

3) BLOOD TESTING: Measure and record blood glucose

   _____ Before meals and at bedtime daily.
   _____ Before meals, 2 hours after meals, and at bedtime daily.
   _____ Once weekly with each urine check.

In addition check your blood glucose occasionally during the night if you
suspect hypoglycemia.

4) URINE TESTING: (if you are not measuring blood glucose at home)
   _____ Test your urine four times a day (before meals and bedtime)
          and record results in per cent (%).
   _____ Test your urine for sugar before breakfast daily and record
          results.
   _____ Test your for acetone:
          1) Every morning before breakfast
          2) If urine sugar is 1% or greater or blood sugar is over 250.
          3) If you are ill and unable to eat normally

5) ADJUSTMENTS of insulin dosage to help compensate for normal
variations in insulin requirements [see algorithms page 46].

6) SUPPLEMENTS for sudden or temporary loss of control, for example "a
virus". Use Regular or Actrapid insulin, which is given in addition to
basal insulin dose. Record the supplement dose separately in your log.

   _____ If blood glucose is 200–249 mg/dl: Add _____ Units
                              250–299 mg/dl: Add _____ Units
                              300–349 mg/dl: Add _____ Units
                              350–399 mg/dl: Add _____ Units
                              400–499 mg/dl: Add _____ Units

   _____ If double-void urine sugar is 1%: Add _____ Units
                                         2%: Add _____ Units
                                         3%: Add _____ Units
                                         5%: Add _____ Units

7) DURING UNUSUAL EXERTION have an extra fruit or bread exchange every
   30 to 45 minutes.

Index